WEIGHT GAIN DIET COOKBOOK FOR MEN

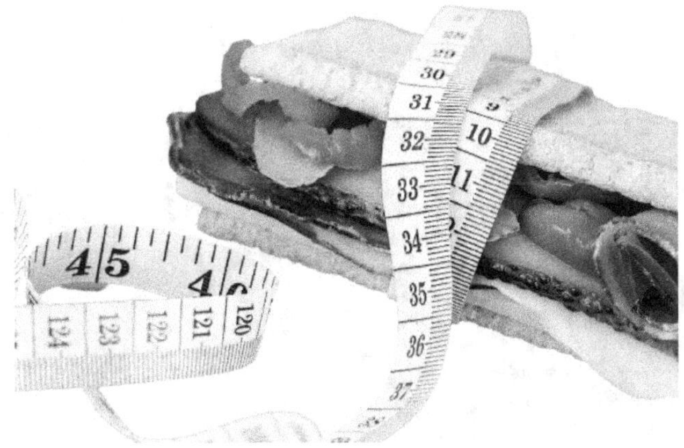

The proven step-by-step guide to weight gain and a healthy life

JERICA R. HOLMES

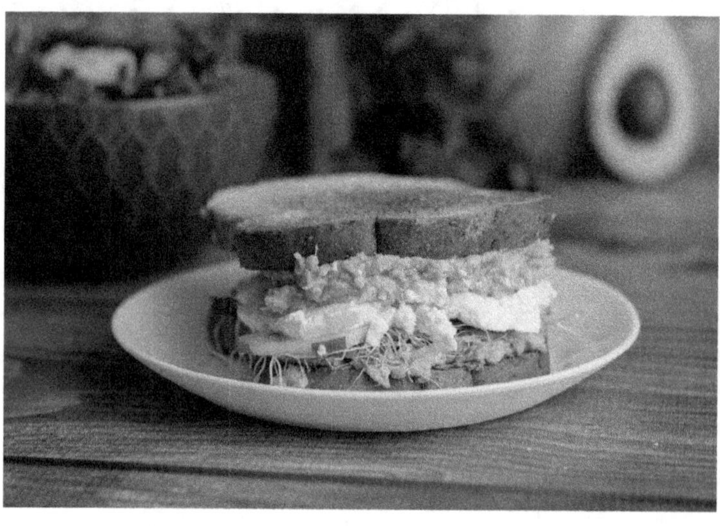

TABLE OF CONTENTS

Snack:

Lunch:

Snack:

Dinner:

Snack:

1500 Calories

Breakfast:

Snack:

Lunch:

Snack:

Dinner:

Snack:

1800 Calories

Breakfast:

Snack:

Lunch:

Snack:

Dinner:

Snack:

CHAPTER 4

HIGH-CALORIE BREAKFAST RECIPES

Avocado and Egg Toast

Banana and peanut butter smoothie

Breakfast burrito

WHY BREAKFAST IS IMPORTANT FOR WEIGHT GAIN

HIGH-CALORIE BREAKFAST RECIPE IDEAS

Banana Oatmeal pancakes

Avocado toast with fried eggs

Breakfast burrito

Blueberry pancakes

Huevos rancheros

Chocolate chip waffles

Fluffy buttermilk pancakes

Biscuits of sausage gravy

Croque monsieur

Sweet potato breakfast hash

Blueberry protein pancakes

Banana nuts muffins

Apples cinnamon oatmeal

Greek yogurt parfait

Blueberry banana pancakes

CHAPTER 5

PROTEIN-RICH MAIN COURSE RECIPES FOR WEIGHT GAIN

Grilled salmon with quinoa and roasted vegetables

Chicken and vegetable stir fry with brown rice

Lentil and vegetable curry

WHY PROTEIN IS IMPORTANT FOR WEIGHT GAIN

PROTEIN-RICH MAIN COURSE RECIPE IDEAS

Grilled chicken breast with roasted vegetables

Baked salmon with asparagus and lemon

Lentil soup with vegetables

Grilled steak with roasted sweet potatoes

Grilled salmon with lemon and herbs

Chicken fajitas

Beef stir fry

Turkey Chili

Grilled chicken with avocado salsa

Tuna salad lettuce wrap

Baked cod with lemon and garlic

Quinoa and black bowl

Grilled steak with chimichurri sause

Lentil and vegetables stir fry

Beef and broccoli stir fry

Chicken and vegetable kabobs

VEGETARIAN AND NON-VEGETARIAN OPTIONS

VEGETARIAN OPTIONS:

Grilled portbello mushroom burger

Vegetarian chili

Caprese salad

Vegetable stir fry

NON-VEGETABLE OPTIONS:

Grilled chicken salad

Baked Salmon with lemon and dill

Chia seed pudding with almond milk

IMPORTANCE OF HEALTHY FATS IN WEIGHT GAIN DIET

HEALTHY FATS RECIPE IDEAS

Avocado toast

Roasted brussels sprouts with bacon and pecans

Salmon and avocado salad

Almond butter banana smoothie

Dark chocolate avocado mousse

Quinoa and avocado salad

Chia seed pudding

Roasted sweet potatoes with tahini sauce

Baked salmon with avocado salsa

Almond butter and banana smoothie

Avocado toast with poached eggs

Roasted cauliflower with tahini dressing

Chocolate chia seed pudding

Grilled shrimp and mango salsa

Spinach salad with strawberries and walnuts.

CHAPTER 8

SMOOTHIES AND SHAKES FOR WEIGHT GAIN

Chocolate peanut butter shake

Mango coconut smoothie

Berry nut smoothies

HOW SMOOTHIES AND SHAKES CAN HELP IN WEIGHT GAIN

RECIPE IDEAS FOR HIGH-CALORIE SMOOTHIES AND SHAKES

Peanut butter banana shake

Chocolate avocado smoothie

Mango coconut shake

Blueberry almond butter smoothie

Oatmeal raisin cookie shake

Nutella banana shake

Chocolate peanut butter banana smoothie

Strawberry coconut shake

Cinnamon roll shake

Almond joy smoothie

Banana nut shake

Blueberry oatmeal shake

Avocado mango smoothie

Peanut butter cup smoothie

Coconut pineapple smoothie

Apple cinnamon oat shake

Chocolate cherry smoothie

Green energy smoothie

Banana nut smoothie

CHAPTER 9

SUPPLEMENTS FOR WEIGHT GAIN

SUPPLEMENTS THAT CAN AID IN WEIGHT GAIN

PROS AND CONS OF USING SUPPLEMENTS

RECOMMENDED DOSAGE AND PRECAUTIONS

INTRODUCTION TO WEIGHT GAIN DIET

Tom a friend of mine had been a skinny guy for as long as he could remember. He had always been self-conscious about his thin frame, especially when he saw his friends who were more muscular and filled out. He had tried everything to gain weight, from drinking protein shakes to lifting weights, but nothing seemed to work.

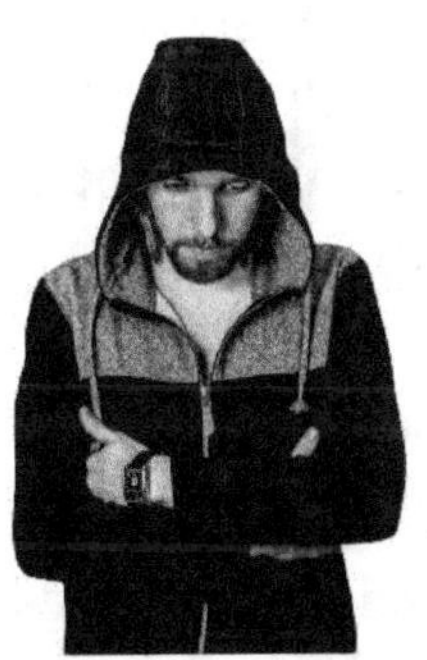

One day, he let out his frustrations by telling how he had been trying to gain weight for as long as he could remember but had not been able to because the weight gain diet manuals he had got for himself had not been able to help him achieve his goals of weight gain.

Since I am a professional dietitian and Nutritionist I told him how he could gain weight by just dieting and some little lifestyle changes. He had come to me for Solutions and there was no way I was going to send him off without one. I told him I was going to arrange a step-by-step guide on how he could gain weight with ease and without fear of side effects like obesity and the rest

When I delivered the guide to him, he immediately began reading it. He was surprised to find that the guide was very detailed and covered everything from diet to exercise routines. He began following the instructions in the guide, starting with the diet plan. He had always thought that he ate enough, but the guide showed him that he needed to consume more calories and protein to gain weight.

Tom started incorporating more high-calorie foods into his diet and even started meal prepping. He also began lifting weights, following the exercise routines provided in this book. He was amazed at how quickly he started seeing results.

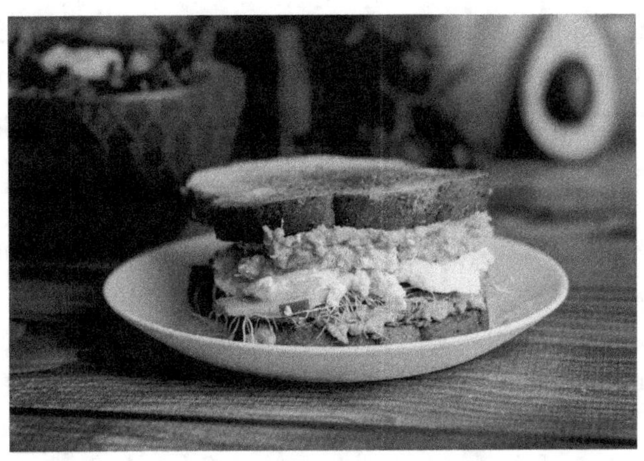

Within a few weeks, Tom began noticing that his clothes were fitting tighter, and his muscles were more defined. He had also gained a few pounds, something he had never been able to achieve before. He was overjoyed and felt more confident than ever.

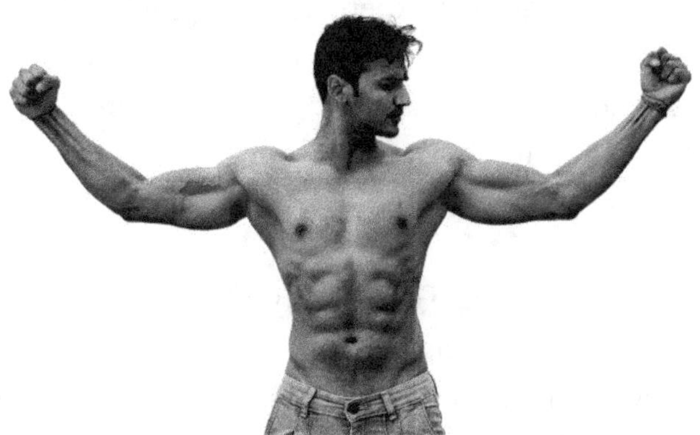

As he continued to follow the plan in the guide, Tom began feeling more energetic and focused. He also noticed that his overall health had improved, with fewer colds and a stronger immune system. His friends and family also noticed the difference and began complimenting him on his physique.

After a few months of following the plan in the book, Tom visited me and by that time he had gained over 20 pounds, and his body had transformed completely. He was no longer the skinny guy he used to be but was now a muscular and confident man. He was grateful to have found reality to his dreams of gaining weight in my guide which had changed his life and helped him achieve his goals.

Tom began recommending my guide to his friends who also struggled with gaining weight. He even started to share his experience and provide tips for others who wanted to gain weight. He knew firsthand how frustrating it was to be skinny and how much it could affect one's confidence and self-esteem.

Tom's life changed completely after he decided to try the book on weight gain. He had achieved what he had been wanting for years and had even become an inspiration to others. The guide not only helped him gain weight but also improved his overall health and well-being. Tom was grateful to have found the book and couldn't imagine where he would be without it.

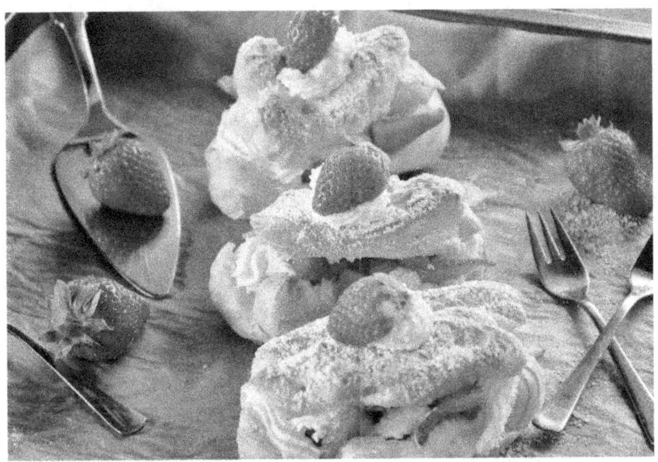

Following the success of Tom's weight gain journey, I decided to combine everything in the guide and additional informations together with a free 10 page meal planner into a single book to help a lot of Men out there who are also tired of going from one book to another in search of ways they can gain weight as this would be the final book that would help them achieve their goals on weight gain.

This weight gain diet cookbook for men is a dietary plan designed to help men gain weight by consuming more calories than their body burns. It is typically recommended for men who are underweight, have a fast metabolism, or are looking to build muscle mass.

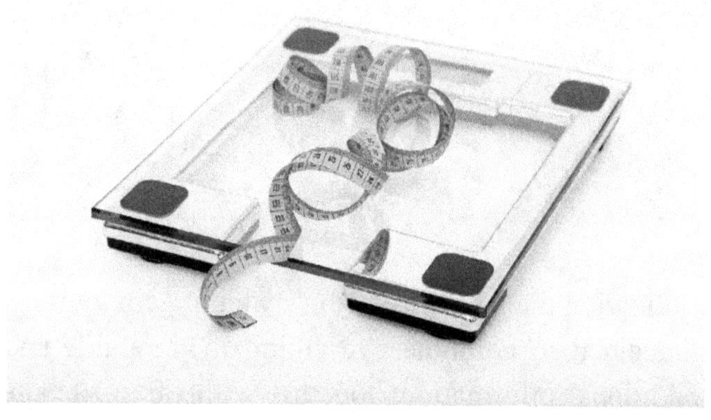

The goal of this weight gain diet cookbook is to provide the body with the necessary nutrients and energy to support weight gain, while maintaining a healthy balance of macronutrients such as carbohydrates, proteins, and fats. The diet typically involves consuming more calories than the body burns, with a focus on nutrient-dense foods such as lean proteins, whole grains, fruits, and vegetables.

In addition to consuming more calories, individuals following a weight gain diet may also need to adjust their exercise routine to include strength training exercises, which can help promote muscle growth and weight gain.

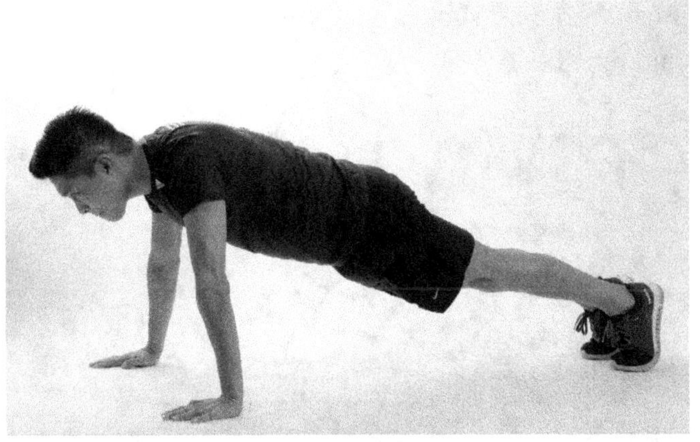

It's important to note that while a weight gain diet can be helpful for individuals looking to gain weight, it's essential to consult a healthcare professional or a registered dietitian before starting any new dietary plan, especially if you have any underlying health conditions or concerns.

In general, a weight gain diet should focus on consuming nutrient-dense, calorie-rich foods. This means avoiding empty calories from processed foods and sugary beverages, and instead opting for whole foods that are rich in vitamins, minerals, and other essential nutrients.

Some examples of nutrient-dense foods that can support weight gain include:

Lean proteins such as chicken, turkey, fish, eggs, and lean beef

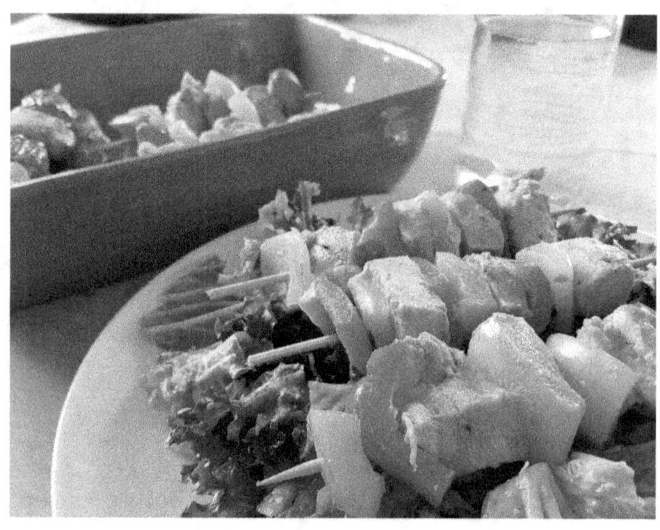

Whole grains such as brown rice, quinoa, oats, and whole wheat bread

Healthy fats such as nuts, seeds, avocado, and olive oil

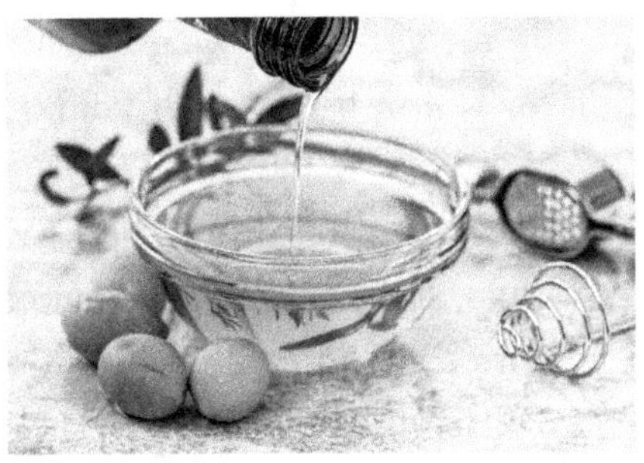

Fruits and vegetables, which provide important vitamins and minerals while also adding fiber to the diet

Dairy products such as milk, cheese, and yogurt, which can provide additional protein and calories.

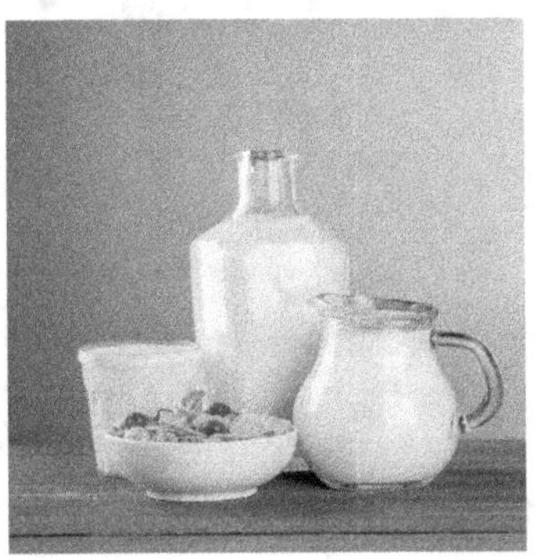

In addition to focusing on nutrient-dense foods, individuals following a weight gain diet may also need to increase their calorie intake by consuming larger portion sizes or adding calorie-dense foods to their meals. This might include adding healthy oils

or nut butters to meals, or snacking on calorie-dense foods like dried fruit or trail mix throughout the day.

It's important to keep in mind that weight gain should be gradual and healthy, and that consuming too many calories or unhealthy foods can have negative health consequences. A healthcare professional or registered dietitian can help individuals determine the appropriate calorie intake and make personalized recommendations for a healthy weight gain diet.

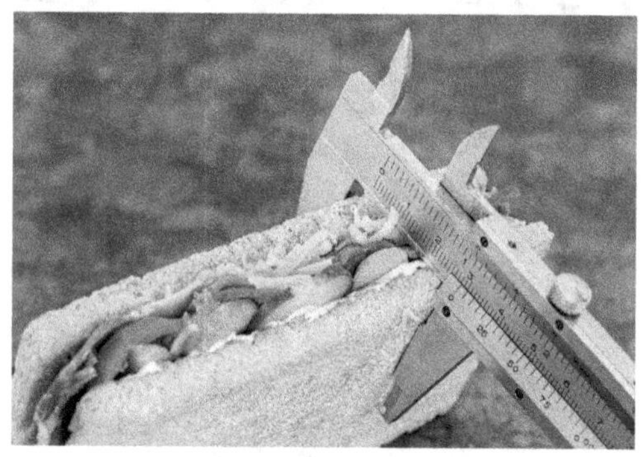

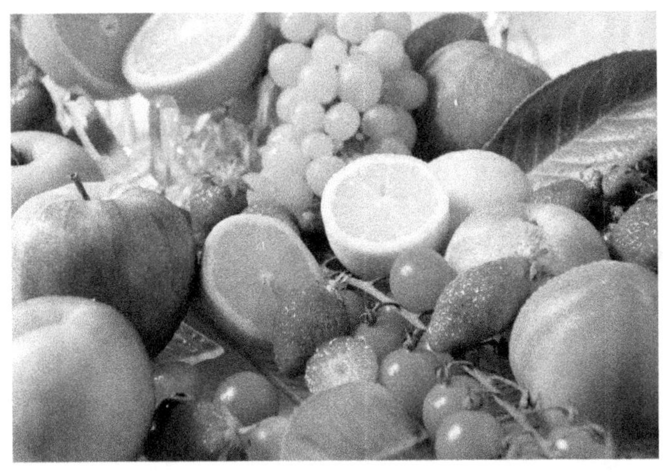

CHAPTER 1

WHY WEIGHT GAIN CAN BE DIFFICULT FOR SOME MEN

There are a variety of reasons why some men may struggle to gain weight, including:

1. Genetics: Genetics play a significant role in determining a person's body type, metabolism, and weight distribution. Some people may have a naturally higher metabolism or a leaner body type, which can make it more difficult for them to gain weight.

2. Hormones: Hormones such as testosterone and growth hormone can also impact weight gain. Men who have low levels of these hormones may find it harder to put on weight and muscle mass.

3. Diet: Diet plays a critical role in weight gain. Men who struggle to gain weight may not be consuming enough calories or consuming the right types of foods to support weight gain. A balanced diet that includes plenty of protein, healthy fats, and complex carbohydrates can help support weight gain.

4. Physical activity: Men who are highly active or engage in intense physical activity may burn more calories, making it harder for them to gain weight. Reducing the amount of cardio or high-intensity exercise and focusing on strength training can help build muscle mass and support weight gain.

5. Medical conditions: Certain medical conditions, such as hyperthyroidism, can also make it difficult for men to gain weight. If a man is struggling to gain weight despite a healthy diet and lifestyle changes, he should talk to his doctor to rule out any underlying medical issues.

6. Stress and sleep: Chronic stress and lack of sleep can also contribute to difficulty gaining weight. When the body is stressed or tired, it releases cortisol, a hormone that can impact appetite and metabolism. Getting enough restful sleep and managing stress through relaxation techniques like meditation or yoga can help support weight gain.

7. Age: As men age, their metabolism slows down, and they may lose muscle mass, making it harder to gain weight. This can be due to hormonal changes, a decrease in physical activity, or a decrease in calorie intake. As a result, older men may need to adjust their diet and exercise routine to support weight gain. Consuming more protein, engaging in

strength training, and reducing the amount of cardio exercise can all be beneficial for older men who are struggling to gain weight.

8. Underlying medical conditions: Certain medical conditions can make it difficult for men to gain weight. For example, gastrointestinal disorders such as celiac disease, inflammatory bowel disease, or chronic diarrhea can affect nutrient absorption and make it harder to gain weight. In addition, certain medications, such as those used to treat depression or ADHD, can decrease appetite and lead to weight loss. Men who are experiencing unexplained weight loss or who are struggling to gain weight despite a healthy diet and lifestyle should talk to their doctor to rule out any underlying medical issues.

9. Eating disorders: Although eating disorders are often associated with women, they can affect men as well. Men with eating disorders, such as anorexia or bulimia, may have an intense fear of gaining weight and may engage in restrictive eating or purging behaviors. These behaviors can lead to significant weight loss and malnutrition, making it difficult for men to gain weight. If a man is experiencing symptoms of an eating disorder, he should seek professional help from a therapist or physician who specializes in eating disorders.

10. Lifestyle factors: Certain lifestyle factors can make it difficult for men to gain weight, such as smoking or excessive alcohol consumption. Smoking can decrease appetite and may increase metabolism, making it harder to gain weight. Similarly, excessive alcohol consumption can interfere with nutrient absorption and may lead to weight loss. Reducing or eliminating these lifestyle factors can help support weight gain.

BENEFITS OF GAINING WEIGHT IN A HEALTHY WAY

Gaining weight in a healthy way can have several benefits, including:

1. Increased muscle mass: Gaining weight through exercise and strength training can increase muscle mass, which can improve overall strength and physical performance.

2. Improved immune system: Eating a balanced diet with enough nutrients can boost the immune system and improve overall health.

3. Increased energy levels: A healthy weight gain can provide the body with enough energy to perform daily tasks and exercise.

4. Improved self-esteem: Achieving a healthy weight can improve self-confidence and self-esteem.

5. Reduced risk of disease: Gaining weight in a healthy way can reduce the risk of developing chronic diseases such as heart disease, diabetes, and some types of cancer.

6. Improved mental health: Gaining weight in a healthy way can also improve mental health by reducing stress, anxiety, and depression.

7. Improved digestion: Eating a balanced diet can improve digestion and reduce digestive problems such as constipation and bloating.

8. Improved hormonal balance: Gaining weight in a healthy way can help balance hormones in the body, particularly for individuals who have previously been underweight or experiencing hormonal imbalances. Adequate intake of healthy fats, proteins, and carbohydrates can support hormone production and regulation.

9. Improved reproductive health: Gaining weight in a healthy way can improve reproductive health for both men and women. Adequate body fat is necessary for the proper functioning of reproductive organs and hormone production. In women, gaining weight can improve menstrual regularity and increase the chances of ovulation. In men, gaining weight can improve sperm quality and quantity.

10. Improved bone health: Gaining weight in a healthy way can also improve bone health, particularly for individuals who were previously underweight. Adequate intake of calcium, vitamin D, and other nutrients can strengthen bones, reducing the risk of fractures and osteoporosis later in life.

Overall, gaining weight in a healthy way can lead to improved physical, mental, and emotional health, and reduce the risk of developing chronic diseases.

KEY PRINCIPLES OF A WEIGHT GAIN DIET

A weight gain diet is designed to help individuals increase their body weight and muscle mass. The key principles of a weight gain diet include:

1. Caloric Surplus: To gain weight, you need to consume more calories than your body burns in a day. This is known as a caloric surplus, and it's essential for gaining weight. Calculate your daily caloric needs using an online calculator, and aim to consume 300-500 more calories per day than your maintenance level.

2. Macronutrient Balance: Your diet should include a balance of macronutrients, which are carbohydrates, proteins, and fats. A good starting point for a weight gain diet is a ratio of 40% carbohydrates, 30% protein, and 30% fat. However, this can vary depending on individual needs and preferences.

3. Protein Intake: Protein is essential for building and repairing muscles, so it's important to consume enough of it in your diet. Aim for 1.5-2 grams of protein per kilogram of body weight per day.

4. Healthy Fats: Healthy fats, such as those found in nuts, seeds, avocados, and fish, are an important part of a weight gain diet. They provide energy and support hormone production.

5. Carbohydrates: Carbohydrates provide energy for your body, and are an important part of a weight

gain diet. Focus on complex carbohydrates such as whole grains, fruits, and vegetables, rather than simple sugars.

6. Meal Frequency: Eating frequently throughout the day can help ensure that you're consuming enough calories to gain weight. Aim for 3-4 larger meals, with 2-3 snacks in between.

7. Resistance Training: In addition to diet, resistance training is important for building muscle mass. Aim to lift weights or engage in other resistance training exercises at least 2-3 times per week.

8. Patience and Consistency: Gaining weight takes time and consistency. Stick to your diet and exercise plan, and be patient with the results. It's important to focus on making sustainable lifestyle changes rather than quick fixes.

CHAPTER 2

UNDERSTANDING MACRONUTRIENTS FOR WEIGHT GAIN

To gain weight, men need to consume more calories than they burn through physical activity and daily functions. Macronutrients, such as protein, carbohydrates, and fats, are essential for weight gain as they provide energy and help build muscle. Here is a breakdown of how these macronutrients can help with weight gain for men:

Protein: Protein is important for building and repairing muscle tissue, which is necessary for gaining weight. Men who want to gain weight should aim to consume at least 1 gram of protein per pound of body weight each day. Good sources of protein include lean meats, poultry, fish, eggs, dairy products, beans, and nuts.

Carbohydrates: Carbohydrates provide the body with energy and are essential for weight gain. Men who want to gain weight should aim to consume complex carbohydrates, such as whole grains, vegetables, and fruits. Simple carbohydrates, such as sugar and processed foods, should be limited as they can cause spikes in blood sugar and lead to weight gain in the form of fat.

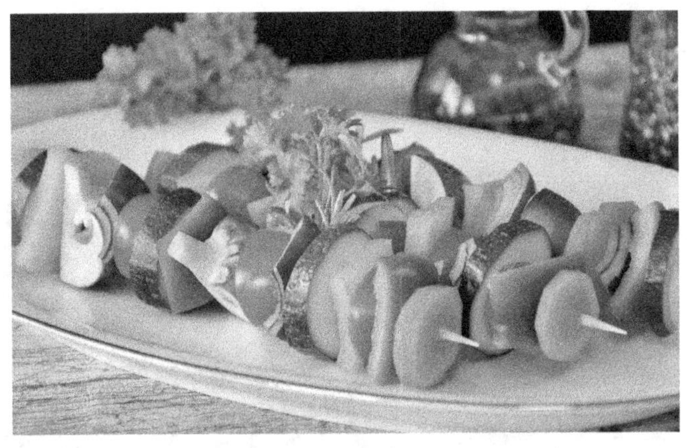

Fats: Fats are important for overall health and can help men gain weight by providing extra calories. However, it is important to choose healthy fats, such as those found in nuts, seeds, avocados, and fatty fish, rather than unhealthy fats found in fried foods and processed snacks.

In addition to the three macronutrients mentioned earlier, there is also a fourth macronutrient - fiber - which is important for overall health and weight gain.

Fibre: Fiber is a type of carbohydrate that cannot be digested by the body, but it is important for digestive health and can help with weight gain. High-fiber foods, such as fruits, vegetables, whole grains, and legumes, can help you feel fuller for longer, which can prevent overeating and promote weight gain in a healthy way.

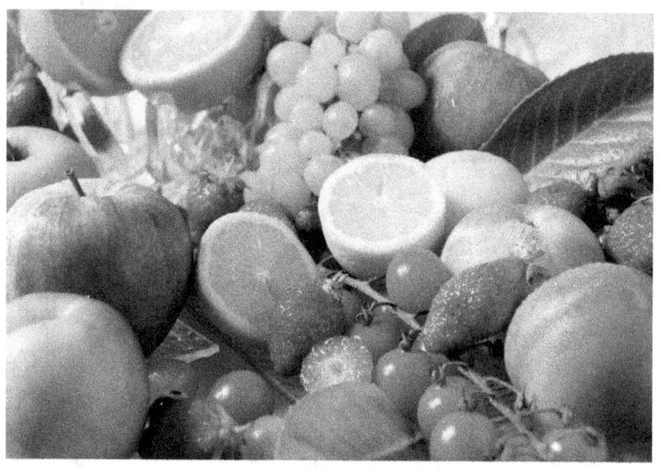

It is important to note that simply consuming more calories does not necessarily mean healthy weight gain. Eating a balanced diet with nutrient-dense foods is essential for overall health and sustainable weight gain. Additionally, regular exercise and adequate sleep are also important factors in achieving healthy weight gain.

What are macronutrients (protein, carbohydrates, and fats)?

Macronutrients are the three main categories of nutrients that are essential for human health and survival: protein, carbohydrates, and fats.

Protein: Protein is made up of amino acids and is an essential macronutrient for building and repairing tissues, enzymes, hormones, and antibodies. Protein is also used as a source of energy when carbohydrate and fat stores are depleted.

Amino acids are the building blocks of protein and there are 20 different types, 9 of which are considered essential because the body cannot produce them on its own and they must be obtained through the diet.

Sources of protein include animal products such as meat, fish, poultry, eggs, and dairy, as well as plant-based sources such as legumes, nuts, and seeds.

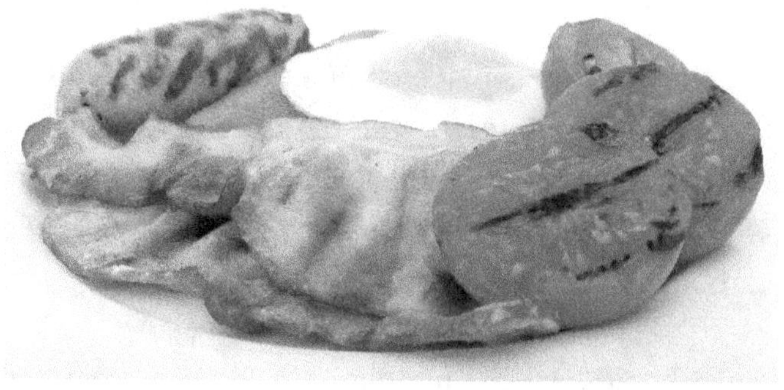

Carbohydrates: Carbohydrates are an essential macronutrient and a primary source of energy for the body. There are two types of carbohydrates: simple and complex. Simple carbohydrates are found in foods like fruit, milk, and candy and are broken down quickly by the body for energy.

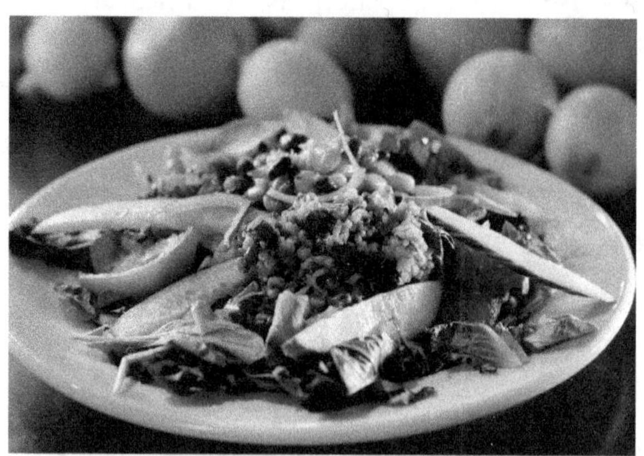

Complex carbohydrates are found in foods like vegetables, beans, and whole grains and are broken down more slowly, providing a longer-lasting source of energy. Carbohydrates are also important for brain function and for providing fuel for exercise.

Fats: Fats are an essential macronutrient that provide the body with energy, help to insulate and protect organs, and aid in the absorption of fat-soluble vitamins.

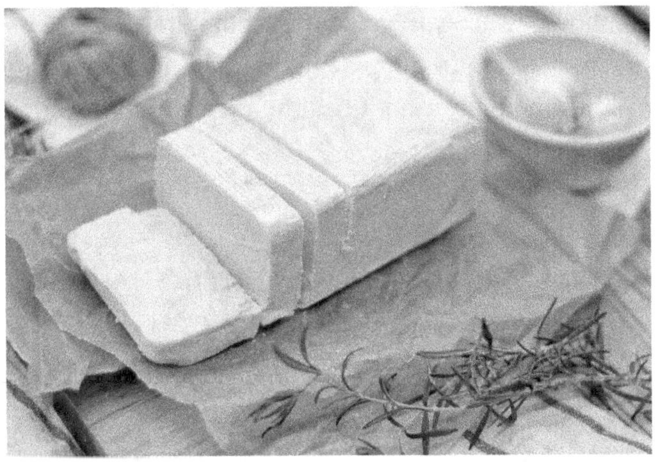

There are three main types of fats: saturated, unsaturated, and trans fats. Saturated fats are typically solid at room temperature and are found in foods like butter, cheese, and fatty meats. Unsaturated fats are typically liquid at room temperature and are found in foods like nuts, seeds, and fish.

Trans fats are a type of unsaturated fat that are artificially created through a process called hydrogenation and are found in many processed foods. It is recommended to limit the intake of saturated and trans fats and to include more sources of healthy unsaturated fats in the diet.

In summary, macronutrients are the three main categories of nutrients that are essential for human health and survival: protein, carbohydrates, and fats. Each macronutrient plays a unique and important role in the body, and a healthy diet should include a balance of all three.

IMPORTANCE OF MACRONUTRIENTS RATIOS FOR WEIGHT GAIN

Macronutrient ratios can play an important role in weight gain for men, as they determine the amount of protein, carbohydrates, and fat in their diet. Here are a few key points to keep in mind:

Calories are key: In order to gain weight, men need to consume more calories than they burn on a daily basis. This is known as a calorie surplus. The specific number of calories needed will depend on factors such as age, height, weight, and activity level.

Protein is important: Protein is essential for building and repairing muscle tissue, which is important for weight gain. Men who are looking to gain weight should aim to consume 1-1.5 grams of protein per pound of body weight per day. This can be obtained from sources such as meat, fish, poultry, eggs, dairy, and plant-based sources such as legumes, tofu, and tempeh.

Carbohydrates provide energy: Carbohydrates are the body's primary source of energy, and are important for fueling workouts and recovery. Men who are looking to gain weight should aim to consume 2-3 grams of carbohydrates per pound of body weight per day. This can be obtained from sources such as whole grains, fruits, vegetables, and starchy vegetables such as potatoes and sweet potatoes.

Fat is also important: While fat often gets a bad rap, it is important for a healthy diet and can help men gain weight. Men who are looking to gain weight should aim to consume 0.5-1 gram of fat per pound of body weight per day. This can be obtained from sources such as nuts, seeds, avocado, olive oil, and fatty fish.

In general, a good macronutrient ratio for weight gain for men is around 40% carbohydrates, 30% protein, and 30% fat. However, it is important to remember that everyone's nutritional needs are different, and that individual factors such as age, weight, height, and activity level should also be taken into account when determining the ideal macronutrient ratio.

It may be helpful to work with a registered dietitian or nutritionist to develop a personalize nutrition plan for weight gain.

RECOMMENDED DAILY INTAKE OF MACRONUTRIENTS FOR MEN

The recommended daily intake of macronutrients for men varies depending on several factors such as age, weight, height, physical activity level, and overall health. However, generally, the following are the recommended daily intake of macronutrients for adult men:

Carbohydrates: 225-325 grams per day, or 45-65% of total daily calorie intake.
Proteins: 56-91 grams per day, or 10-35% of total daily calorie intake.

Fats: 20-35% of total daily calorie intake, with a focus on consuming unsaturated fats, such as those found in fish, nuts, and vegetable oils.

It's essential to note that these recommendations are just general guidelines and that the ideal macronutrient intake for each individual will vary depending on their specific needs and goals. Therefore, it is always best to consult with a healthcare provider or registered dietitian for personalized nutrition advice.

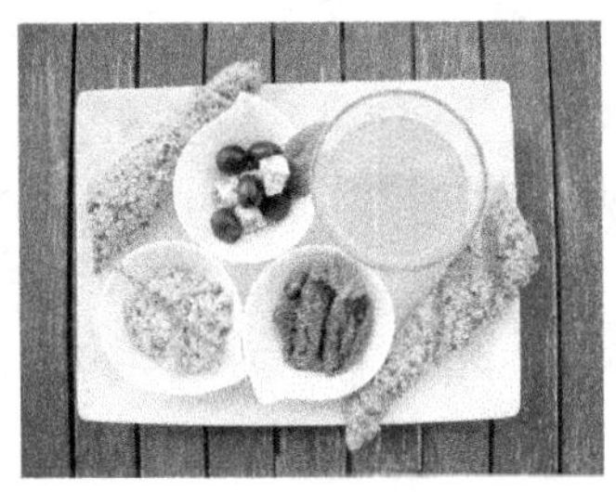

CHAPTER 3

MEAL PLANNING FOR WEIGHT GAIN

If you are looking to gain weight, it's important to consume more calories than you burn. However, it's also important to make sure you are getting enough nutrients and not just consuming empty calories. Here are some tips for meal planning for weight gain:

Focus on nutrient-dense foods: Incorporate plenty of fruits, vegetables, whole grains, lean proteins, and healthy fats into your diet. These foods will provide your body with the necessary vitamins, minerals, and nutrients to support muscle growth and overall health.

Increase calorie intake: In order to gain weight, you need to eat more calories than you burn. Aim for a calorie surplus of 250-500 calories per day.

Eat frequently: Rather than eating three large meals per day, try eating 5-6 smaller meals throughout the day. This will help ensure you are consuming enough calories and nutrients.

Choose calorie-dense foods: Include foods that are high in calories but still nutrient-dense, such as nuts, nut butters, avocados, and dried fruits.

Incorporate protein: Protein is essential for building and repairing muscle tissue. Aim for a minimum of 1 gram of protein per pound of body weight per day.

Don't skip carbs: Carbohydrates provide your body with energy, so it's important to include them in your diet. Choose complex carbs such as whole grains, fruits, and vegetables.

Stay hydrated: Make sure you are drinking plenty of water throughout the day to support digestion, nutrient absorption, and overall health.

SAMPLE MEAL PLAN:

Breakfast:

2 eggs scrambled with spinach and whole wheat toast with avocado
1 cup of Greek yogurt with granola and mixed berries
1 banana

Snack:

Smoothie made with protein powder, banana, almond milk, and peanut butter

Lunch:

Turkey sandwich on whole wheat bread with lettuce, tomato, and avocado
Carrots and hummus
Apple

Snack:

Handful of almonds and a piece of fruit

Dinner:

Grilled salmon with quinoa and roasted vegetables
Salad with mixed greens, cucumber, and tomato
1 slice of whole wheat bread with olive oil and balsamic vinegar for dipping

Snack:

Greek yogurt with honey and mixed berries

Remember, gaining weight takes time and consistency. Stick to your meal plan and stay committed to your fitness routine to see results.

SAMPLE MEAL PLANS FOR DIFFERENT CALORIE NEEDS

Here are some sample meal plans for different calorie needs:

1200 Calories:

Breakfast:

Ze1 cup of oatmeal, 1 medium banana, and 1 tablespoon of peanut butter.

Snack:

1 small apple and 1 tablespoon of almond
butter.

Lunch:

2 cups of mixed greens with 1/2 cup of chickpeas,
1/2 cup of cherry tomatoes, and 2 tablespoons of
balsamic vinaigrette.

Snack:

1/2 cup of sliced cucumber and 2 tablespoons of
hummus.

Dinner:

3 ounces of grilled chicken breast, 1 cup of steamed
broccoli, and 1/2 cup of cooked quinoa.

1500 Calories:

Breakfast:

2 scrambled eggs, 1 slice of whole-grain toast, and 1 medium orange.

Snack:

1 medium pear and 1 ounce of mixed nuts.

Lunch:

1/2 cup of brown rice, 1/2 cup of black beans, 1/2 cup of sliced bell peppers, and 1 tablespoon of salsa.

Snack:

1 small banana and 1 tablespoon of almond butter.

Dinner:

4 ounces of baked salmon, 1 cup of roasted sweet potatoes, and 1 cup of sautéed spinach.

1800 Calories:

Breakfast:

1 cup of Greek yogurt, 1/2 cup of mixed berries, and 1/4 cup of granola.

Snack:

1 small apple and 2 tablespoons of peanut butter.

Lunch:

2 slices of whole-grain bread, 3 ounces of turkey breast, 1 slice of cheddar cheese, and 1/2 cup of baby carrots.

Snack:

1/2 cup of sliced cucumber and 1/4 cup of tzatziki sauce.

Dinner:

5 ounces of grilled flank steak, 1 cup of roasted brussels sprouts, and 1/2 cup of cooked quinoa.

Note: These meal plans are just examples and should be adjusted to meet individual preferences and dietary requirements.

HOW TO BALANCE MACRONUTRIENT IN EACH MEAL

Balancing macronutrients in each meal involves making sure that you consume the right amounts of carbohydrates, proteins, and fats to support your body's needs. Here are some general guidelines for balancing macronutrients in each meal:

Start with protein: Aim to include a source of protein in each meal, such as chicken, fish, tofu, lentils, beans, or eggs. Protein helps to build and repair tissues in your body and keeps you feeling full and satisfied.

Add carbohydrates: Carbohydrates provide your body with energy, so include a source of complex carbohydrates in each meal, such as brown rice, sweet potatoes, quinoa, or whole wheat bread. Complex carbohydrates are also high in fiber, which helps to keep you feeling full and aids in digestion.

Include healthy fats: Healthy fats, such as those found in nuts, seeds, avocado, and olive oil, are important for brain function, hormone production, and overall health. However, it's important to be mindful of portion sizes, as fats are high in calories.

Pay attention to portion sizes: To balance macronutrients in each meal, it's important to pay attention to portion sizes. A general rule of thumb is to aim for a palm-sized portion of protein, a fist-sized portion of complex carbohydrates, and a thumb-sized portion of healthy fats.

Consider your individual needs: Keep in mind that the ideal macronutrient balance for each meal may vary depending on your individual needs and goals. For example, athletes may need more carbohydrates to fuel their workouts, while someone trying to lose weight may need to focus on portion control and reducing their overall calorie intake.

It's important to prioritize whole, nutrient-dense foods in your diet and to aim for a balanced macronutrient intake throughout the day. Consulting with a registered dietitian can also be helpful in determining the optimal macronutrient balance for your individual needs.

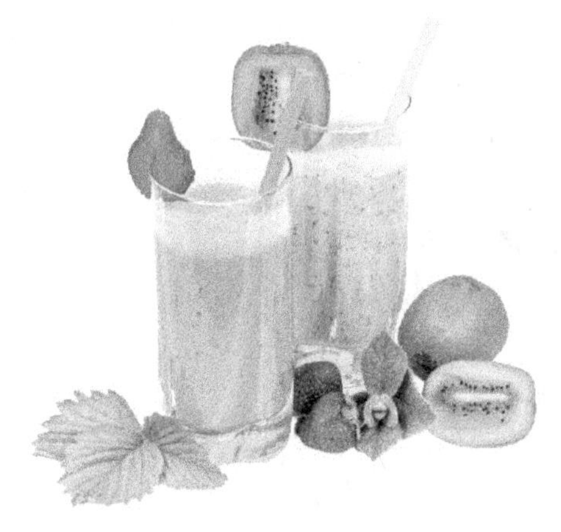

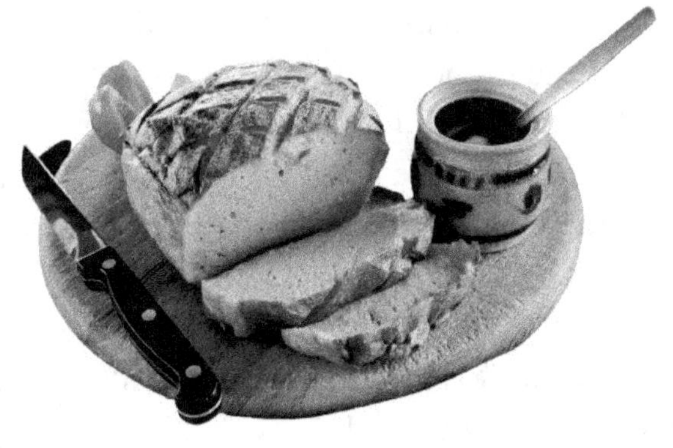

CHAPTER 4

HIGH-CALORIE BREAKFAST RECIPES

Here are three high-calorie breakfast recipes:

AVOCADO AND EGG TOAST

2 slices of whole grain bread
1 ripe avocado
2 eggs
Salt and pepper to taste
1 tbsp olive oil

Instructions:

Preheat the oven to 375°F.
Slice the avocado in half and remove the pit. Mash the flesh in a small bowl with a fork and season with salt and pepper.
Toast the bread until golden brown.
Heat the olive oil in a non-stick skillet over medium heat. Crack the eggs into the skillet and cook until the whites are set but the yolks are still runny.
Spread the mashed avocado on the toasted bread and top with the fried eggs. Season with additional salt and pepper if desired.

Nutrition information (per serving):

Calories: 502
Protein: 19g
Carbs: 37g
Fat: 33g
Fiber: 14g
Sugar: 3g

BANANA AND PEANUT BUTTER SMOOTHIE

1 ripe banana
2 tbsp natural peanut butter
1 cup unsweetened almond milk
1 tbsp honey
1 scoop vanilla protein powder (optional)

Instructions:

Blend all ingredients in a blender until smooth.
Pour into a glass and enjoy immediately.

Nutrition information (per serving):

Calories: 425
Protein: 20g
Carbs: 46g
Fat: 19g
Fiber: 7g
Sugar: 25g

BREAKFAST BURRITO

2 large flour tortillas
4 large eggs
1/2 cup black beans
1/2 cup cooked brown rice

1/4 cup grated cheddar cheese
Salt and pepper to taste
1 tbsp olive oil

Instructions:

Heat the olive oil in a non-stick skillet over medium heat.
Crack the eggs into the skillet and scramble until cooked through.
Add the black beans and cooked rice to the skillet and stir until heated through.
Season with salt and pepper.
Warm the tortillas in the microwave for 30 seconds.
Divide the egg mixture between the two tortillas and top with grated cheddar cheese.
Roll up the tortillas and serve.

Nutrition Information (Per Serving):

Calories: 770
Protein: 35g
Carbs: 78g
Fat: 33g
Fiber: 10g
Sugar: 1g

WHY BREAKFAST IS IMPORTANT FOR WEIGHT GAIN

Breakfast is important for weight gain for men because it kickstarts the body's metabolism after a night of fasting. When you skip breakfast, your body remains in a state of "resting" metabolism and burns fewer calories throughout the day. This can make it more difficult to gain weight, as your body is not using as much energy.

Furthermore, a nutritious breakfast can provide the body with the energy and nutrients needed to support weight gain. Eating a balanced breakfast that includes protein, carbohydrates, and healthy fats can help increase muscle mass, which can contribute to weight gain.

In addition, skipping breakfast can lead to overeating later in the day, which can lead to weight gain in the form of excess body fat. Eating a filling breakfast can help prevent overeating and control hunger throughout the day, making it easier to maintain a healthy weight.

Overall, breakfast is an important meal for men who are trying to gain weight, as it can support the body's metabolism, provide necessary nutrients, and help prevent overeating later in the day.

HIGH-CALORIE BREAKFAST RECIPE IDEAS

BANANA OATMEAL PANCAKES

Ingredients:

1 ripe banana
1/2 cup rolled oats
1 egg
1/2 teaspoon baking powder
1/4 teaspoon cinnamon
1 tablespoon maple syrup
1 tablespoon butter

Instructions:

In a bowl, mash the banana with a fork.
Add the oats, egg, baking powder, cinnamon, and maple syrup to the bowl. Mix well.
Heat the butter in a non-stick pan over medium heat.
Pour the pancake batter into the pan and cook for 2-3 minutes on each side, or until golden brown.
Serve hot with additional maple syrup, if desired.

Nutrition Information (per serving):

Calories: 435
Protein: 10g
Fat: 18g

Carbohydrates: 62g

AVOCADO TOAST WITH FRIED EGG

Ingredients:

1 slice of whole wheat bread
1/2 avocado
1 egg
1 teaspoon olive oil
Salt and pepper to taste

Instructions:

Toast the bread.
Mash the avocado in a bowl.
In a non-stick pan, heat the olive oil over medium heat.
Crack the egg into the pan and cook until the whites are set and the yolk is still runny.
Spread the mashed avocado on the toast and sprinkle with salt and pepper.
Place the fried egg on top of the avocado toast.

Nutrition Information (per serving):

Calories: 368
Protein: 13g
Fat: 27g

Carbohydrates: 20g

BREAKFAST BURRITO

Ingredients:

2 large eggs
2 slices of bacon
1/4 cup shredded cheddar cheese
1/4 cup diced tomatoes
1/4 cup diced onion
1/4 cup diced green bell pepper
1/2 avocado, diced
2 flour tortillas
Salt and pepper to taste

Instructions:

Cook the bacon in a non-stick pan over medium heat until crispy. Remove from pan and crumble.
In the same pan, sauté the onion and bell pepper until softened.
Add the eggs to the pan and scramble until cooked through.
Warm the tortillas in the microwave or on a griddle.
Divide the scrambled eggs, bacon, cheese, tomatoes, onion, bell pepper, and avocado between the tortillas.
Roll up the tortillas, tucking in the sides, and serve.

Nutrition Information (per serving):

Calories: 590
Protein: 26g
Fat: 39g
Carbohydrates: 33g

BLUEBERRY PANCAKES

Ingredients:

1 cup all-purpose flour
1 tablespoon sugar
1 teaspoon baking powder
1/2 teaspoon baking soda
1/4 teaspoon salt
1 cup milk
1 egg
2 tablespoons butter, melted
1 cup blueberries

Instructions:

In a large bowl, whisk together the flour, sugar, baking powder, baking soda, and salt.
In a separate bowl, whisk together the milk, egg, and melted butter.

Pour the wet ingredients into the dry ingredients and stir until just combined.

Fold in the blueberries.

Heat a non-stick pan over medium heat and grease with cooking spray or butter.

Pour 1/4 cup of batter onto the pan for each pancake.

Cook for 2-3 minutes on each side, or until golden brown.

Serve hot with butter and maple syrup.

Nutrition Information (per serving):

Calories: 360
Protein: 9g
Fat: 11g
Carbohydrates: 56g

HUEVOS RANCHEROS

Ingredients:

2 large eggs
2 corn tortillas
1/4 cup refried beans
1/4 cup shredded cheddar cheese
1/4 cup salsa
1 tablespoon olive oil
Salt and pepper to taste

Instructions:

Warm the tortillas in a dry skillet or in the microwave.
Heat the refried beans in a small saucepan.
In a separate non-stick pan, heat the olive oil over medium heat.
Crack the eggs into the pan and cook until the whites are set and the yolks are still runny.
Place the warmed tortillas on plates and spread the refried beans on top.
Place the fried eggs on top of the beans and sprinkle with shredded cheese.
Spoon the salsa over the top.
Serve hot.

Nutrition Information (per serving):

Calories: 423
Protein: 20g
Fat: 24g
Carbohydrates: 33g

CHOCOLATE CHIP WAFFLES

Ingredients:

1 1/2 cups all-purpose flour

2 tablespoons sugar
2 teaspoons baking powder
1/2 teaspoon baking soda
1/4 teaspoon salt
1 1/4 cups milk
2 large eggs
1/4 cup vegetable oil
1/2 cup mini chocolate chips

Instructions:

In a large bowl, whisk together the flour, sugar, baking powder, baking soda, and salt.
In a separate bowl, whisk together the milk, eggs, and vegetable oil.
Pour the wet ingredients into the dry ingredients and stir until just combined.
Fold in the chocolate chips.
Preheat a waffle iron and spray with cooking spray.
Pour 1/2 cup of batter onto the waffle iron and cook according to manufacturer's instructions.
Serve hot with butter and syrup.

Nutrition Information (per serving):

Calories: 528
Protein: 11g
Fat: 27g
Carbohydrates: 63g

FLUFFY BUTTERMILK PANCAKES

Ingredients:

1 1/2 cups all-purpose flour
3 1/2 teaspoons baking powder
1 teaspoon salt
1 tablespoon white sugar
1 1/4 cups buttermilk
1 egg
3 tablespoons butter, melted
Cooking spray or butter for greasing the pan

Instructions:

In a large bowl, whisk together the flour, baking powder, salt, and sugar.
In a separate bowl, whisk together the buttermilk, egg, and melted butter.
Pour the wet ingredients into the dry ingredients and stir until just combined.
Heat a non-stick pan over medium heat and grease with cooking spray or butter.
Pour 1/4 cup of batter onto the pan for each pancake.
Cook for 2-3 minutes on each side, or until golden brown.
Serve hot with butter and maple syrup.

Nutrition Information (per serving):

Calories: 153
Protein: 4g
Fat: 5g
Carbohydrates: 22g

BISCUITS AND SAUSAGE GRAVY

Ingredients:

For the Biscuits:

2 cups all-purpose flour
1 tablespoon baking powder
1 teaspoon salt
1/2 cup cold unsalted butter, cut into small cubes
3/4 cup milk

For the Sausage Gravy:

1 pound breakfast sausage
1/4 cup all-purpose flour
2 cups milk
Salt and pepper to taste

Instructions:

Preheat the oven to 425°F (218°C).

In a large bowl, whisk together the flour, baking powder, and salt.

Using a pastry blender or your fingers, cut the cold butter into the flour mixture until it resembles coarse crumbs.

Add the milk and stir until the dough just comes together.

Turn the dough out onto a lightly floured surface and knead gently for 1-2 minutes.

Roll out the dough to 1/2-inch thickness and cut into rounds using a biscuit cutter.

Place the biscuits on a baking sheet lined with parchment paper and bake for 12-15 minutes, or until golden brown.

For the Sausage Gravy:

In a large skillet over medium-high heat, cook the breakfast sausage until browned and cooked through, breaking it up into small pieces as it cooks.

Sprinkle the flour over the sausage and stir to combine.

Gradually pour in the milk, stirring constantly, and continue to cook until the mixture thickens and comes to a simmer.

Reduce the heat to low and let the gravy simmer for 2-3 minutes, stirring occasionally.

Season with salt and pepper to taste.

To Serve:

Split the warm biscuits in half and place them on plates.
Spoon the sausage gravy over the biscuits.
Serve hot.

Nutrition Information (per serving):

Calories: 563
Protein: 18g
Fat: 37g
Carbohydrates: 40g

CROQUE MONSIEUR

Ingredients:

4 slices of bread (white or sourdough)
4 slices of ham
4 slices of Swiss cheese
2 tablespoons unsalted butter
2 tablespoons all-purpose flour
1 cup milk
Salt and pepper to taste
1/4 cup grated Parmesan cheese

Instructions:

Preheat the broiler to high.

Toast the bread slices and place them on a baking sheet.

Top each slice with a slice of ham and a slice of Swiss cheese.

In a saucepan, melt the butter over medium heat.

Add the flour and whisk constantly for 1-2 minutes, until the mixture is smooth and bubbling.

Gradually whisk in the milk and continue to whisk until the mixture thickens and comes to a simmer.

Remove the saucepan from the heat and season with salt and pepper to taste.

Spoon the sauce over the ham and cheese on each slice of bread.

Sprinkle the grated Parmesan cheese over the sauce.

Broil the Croque Monsieurs for 2-3 minutes, or until the cheese is melted and bubbly.

Serve hot.

Nutrition Information (per serving):

Calories: 416
Protein: 23g
Fat: 24g
Carbohydrates: 25g

SWEET POTATO BREAKFAST HASH

Ingredients:

2 tablespoons olive oil
2 medium sweet potatoes, peeled and diced
1 red bell pepper, seeded and diced
1 small onion, diced
1 teaspoon smoked paprika
1/2 teaspoon garlic powder
Salt and pepper to taste
4 large eggs

Instructions:

In a large skillet, heat the olive oil over medium-high heat.
Add the sweet potatoes, red bell pepper, and onion to the skillet.
Sprinkle the smoked paprika, garlic powder, salt, and pepper over the vegetables.
Cook, stirring occasionally, until the sweet potatoes are tender and lightly browned, about 15 minutes.
Using a spoon, make 4 wells in the sweet potato mixture.
Crack an egg into each well.
Reduce the heat to medium and cover the skillet.
Cook until the eggs are set to your liking, about 5-7 minutes.
Serve hot.

Nutrition Information (per serving):

Calories: 307
Protein: 10g
Fat: 18g
Carbohydrates: 28g

BLUEBERRY PROTEIN PANCAKES

Ingredients:

1 cup rolled oats
1/2 cup low-fat cottage cheese
1/2 cup blueberries
2 eggs
1/2 teaspoon baking powder
1/4 teaspoon salt
1/2 teaspoon vanilla extract
1 tablespoon honey

Instructions:

In a blender, combine the rolled oats, cottage cheese, blueberries, eggs, baking powder, salt, vanilla extract, and honey.
Blend until the mixture is smooth.
Heat a non-stick skillet over medium heat.
Pour 1/4 cup of the pancake batter into the skillet for each pancake.

Cook until bubbles form on the surface of the pancake and the edges are set, about 2-3 minutes.
Flip the pancake and cook for another minute or until lightly browned.
Repeat with the remaining batter.
Serve hot with additional blueberries and maple syrup, if desired.

Nutrition Information (per serving):

Calories: 334
Protein: 20g
Fat: 8g
Carbohydrates: 45g

BANANA NUT MUFFINS

Ingredients:

2 cups all-purpose flour
1 teaspoon baking powder
1 teaspoon baking soda
1/2 teaspoon salt
1/2 cup unsalted butter, softened
3/4 cup brown sugar
2 large eggs
1 teaspoon vanilla extract
1 cup mashed ripe bananas (about 2 bananas)
1/2 cup chopped walnuts

Instructions:

Preheat the oven to 350°F (180°C).
In a bowl, whisk together the flour, baking powder, baking soda, and salt.
In a separate bowl, using an electric mixer, beat the butter and brown sugar together until light and fluffy.
Beat in the eggs, one at a time, followed by the vanilla extract.
Add the mashed bananas and mix until well combined.
Gradually add the flour mixture to the banana mixture and mix until just combined.
Stir in the chopped walnuts.
Line a muffin tin with paper liners.
Spoon the batter into the muffin cups, filling them about 2/3 full.
Bake for 20-25 minutes, or until a toothpick inserted in the center of a muffin comes out clean.
Cool the muffins in the tin for 5 minutes, then transfer them to a wire rack to cool completely.

Nutrition Information (per muffin):

Calories: 275
Protein: 4g
Fat: 13g

Carbohydrates: 36g

APPLE CINNAMON OATMEAL

Ingredients:

1 cup rolled oats
2 cups water
1/2 cup milk
1/4 teaspoon salt
1 apple, peeled, cored, and chopped
1/2 teaspoon cinnamon
1 tablespoon honey
1/4 cup chopped walnuts

Instructions:

In a saucepan, bring the water to a boil.
Add the rolled oats and salt to the saucepan and reduce the heat to low.
Cook, stirring occasionally, for about 5 minutes or until the oats are tender and the mixture has thickened.
Add the milk to the saucepan and stir to combine.
Add the chopped apple, cinnamon, and honey to the saucepan and stir to combine.
Cook the oatmeal for an additional 2-3 minutes or until the apple is tender.
Divide the oatmeal among four bowls.

Sprinkle the chopped walnuts over the oatmeal.
Serve hot.

Nutrition Information (per serving):

Calories: 249
Protein: 8g
Fat: 9g
Carbohydrates: 37g

GREEK YOGURT PARFAIT

Ingredients:

1 cup plain Greek yogurt
1/2 cup granola
1/2 cup mixed berries (such as strawberries, blueberries, and raspberries)
1 tablespoon honey

Instructions:

In a bowl, mix together the Greek yogurt and honey.
Layer the yogurt mixture, granola, and mixed berries in a tall glass or jar.
Repeat the layers until the glass or jar is filled to the top.
Serve immediately.

Nutrition Information (per serving):

Calories: 311
Protein: 18g
Fat: 7g
Carbohydrates: 46g

BLUEBERRY BANANA PANCAKES

Ingredients:

1 cup all-purpose flour
1 tablespoon sugar
1 teaspoon baking powder
1/2 teaspoon baking soda
1/4 teaspoon salt
1 ripe banana, mashed
1 egg
1 cup milk
1 teaspoon vanilla extract
1 cup fresh blueberries
Butter or oil for greasing the pan

Instructions:

In a bowl, whisk together the flour, sugar, baking powder, baking soda, and salt.
In a separate bowl, mix together the mashed banana, egg, milk, and vanilla extract.

Add the wet ingredients to the dry ingredients and mix until just combined.

Gently fold in the blueberries.

Heat a non-stick skillet over medium-high heat.

Grease the skillet with butter or oil.

Using a 1/4 cup measure, pour batter onto the skillet.

Cook for 2-3 minutes or until bubbles form on the surface of the pancake and the edges are set.

Flip the pancake and cook for an additional 1-2 minutes or until the pancake is golden brown.

Repeat with the remaining batter.

Serve hot with butter and maple syrup.

Nutrition Information (per serving):

Calories: 186
Protein: 6g
Fat: 4g
Carbohydrates: 33g

CHAPTER 5

PROTEIN-RICH MAIN COURSE RECIPES FOR WEIGHT GAIN

Here are three protein-rich main course recipes for weight gain with nutritional information:

GRILLED SALMON WITH QUINOA AND ROASTED VEGETABLES

Ingredients:

1 lb salmon fillet
1 cup quinoa
2 cups mixed vegetables (such as bell peppers, zucchini, and onion)
2 tbsp olive oil
Salt and pepper to taste

Instructions:

Preheat the oven to 400°F.
Cook the quinoa according to package

instructions.

Toss the mixed vegetables with 1 tbsp of olive oil, salt, and pepper. Roast them in the oven for 20-25 minutes or until tender.

Brush the salmon fillet with the remaining olive oil and season with salt and pepper.

Grill the salmon over medium-high heat for about 5-6 minutes on each side or until cooked through.

Serve the grilled salmon with the cooked quinoa and roasted vegetables.

Nutritional information (per serving):

Calories: 490
Protein: 36g
Carbohydrates: 34g
Fat: 23g
Fiber: 6g

CHICKEN AND VEGETABLE STIR FRY WITH BROWN RICE

Ingredients:

1 lb boneless, skinless chicken breast, cut into bite-sized pieces
2 cups mixed vegetables (such as broccoli, carrots, and bell peppers)
1 cup brown rice
2 tbsp soy sauce

2 tbsp honey
1 tbsp sesame oil
2 cloves garlic, minced
1 tsp ginger, minced
Salt and pepper to taste

Instructions:

Cook the brown rice according to package instructions.

In a small bowl, whisk together the soy sauce, honey, sesame oil, garlic, ginger, salt, and pepper.

Heat a large skillet over high heat. Add the chicken and stir-fry until browned and cooked through, about 5-7 minutes.

Add the mixed vegetables and continue stir-frying for an additional 3-4 minutes, or until the vegetables are tender.

Pour the sauce over the chicken and vegetables and stir to coat.

Serve the stir-fry with the cooked brown rice.

Nutritional information (per serving):

Calories: 502
Protein: 34g
Carbohydrates: 65g
Fat: 9g
Fiber: 6g

LENTIL AND VEGETABLE CURRY

Ingredients:

1 cup lentils
2 cups mixed vegetables (such as sweet potato, cauliflower, and spinach)
1 can coconut milk
2 tbsp curry powder
2 cloves garlic, minced
1 tbsp ginger, minced
Salt and pepper to taste

Instructions:

Rinse and drain the lentils. Cook them according to package instructions.
While the lentils are cooking, chop the mixed vegetables into bite-sized pieces.
In a large pot, heat the coconut milk over medium heat. Add the curry powder, garlic, ginger, salt, and pepper. Stir to combine.
Add the mixed vegetables to the pot and stir to coat with the curry sauce. Simmer for 15-20 minutes or until the vegetables are tender.
When the lentils are cooked, drain any excess water and add them to the pot with the vegetables. Stir to combine and cook for an additional 5 minutes.

Serve the lentil and vegetable curry over rice or with naan bread.

Nutritional information (per serving):

Calories: 459
Protein: 20g
Carbohydrates: 50g
Fat: 12g
Fiber: 7g

WHY PROTEIN IS IMPORTANT FOR WEIGHT GAIN

Protein is an essential nutrient that plays a critical role in building, repairing, and maintaining tissues in the body, including muscle tissue. When you are trying to gain weight, increasing your protein intake can help you build muscle mass and support your body's overall growth and development.

Here are some ways that protein is important for weight gain:

Muscle growth: When you engage in weight training or other forms of resistance exercise, your muscles undergo small amounts of damage. Protein is necessary for repairing and rebuilding these damaged muscle fibers, which leads to muscle growth and increased strength.

Increased calorie burn: Protein has a higher thermic effect than other macronutrients like carbohydrates and fats, which means that your body burns more calories digesting and metabolizing protein than it does with other nutrients. This increased calorie burn can help support weight gain by boosting your overall calorie intake.

Reduced muscle breakdown: During periods of calorie restriction or weight loss, your body may break down muscle tissue for energy. Adequate protein intake can help prevent this muscle breakdown, ensuring that your body is using stored fat for energy instead of breaking down muscle tissue.

Satiety: Protein is more satiating than other nutrients, meaning that it can help you feel fuller for longer periods, reducing the likelihood of overeating and promoting weight gain.

Overall, protein is essential for weight gain because it supports muscle growth, increases calorie burn, reduces muscle breakdown, and promotes satiety. However, it's important to balance your protein intake with other essential nutrients and to consult with a healthcare professional before making any significant changes to your diet or exercise routine.

PROTEIN-RICH MAIN COURSE RECIPE IDEAS

Some protein-rich main course recipes with instructions and nutrition information:

GRILLED CHICKEN BREAST WITH ROASTED VEGETABLES

Ingredients:

4 boneless, skinless chicken breasts
2 bell peppers
1 onion
2 zucchinis
1 tablespoon olive oil
Salt and pepper to taste

Instructions:

Preheat grill to medium-high heat.
Season the chicken with salt and pepper.
Cut the bell peppers, onion, and zucchinis into bite-sized pieces and toss with olive oil, salt, and pepper.
Grill chicken for 6-7 minutes per side or until cooked through.

Grill the vegetables for 4-5 minutes per side or until tender.

Nutrition information per serving:

Calories: 317
Protein: 38g
Fat: 10g
Carbohydrates: 15g
Fiber: 5g

BAKED SALMON WITH ASPARAGUS AND LEMON

Ingredients:

4 salmon fillets
1 bunch asparagus
1 lemon
1 tablespoon olive oil
Salt and pepper to taste

Instructions:

Preheat oven to 375°F (190°C).
Cut the asparagus into bite-sized pieces and place them on a baking sheet.
Drizzle with olive oil, salt, and pepper.

Season the salmon with salt and pepper and place it on top of the asparagus.

Slice the lemon and place a slice on top of each salmon fillet.

Bake for 12-15 minutes or until the salmon is cooked through.

Nutrition information per serving:

Calories: 347
Protein: 35g
Fat: 21g
Carbohydrates: 6g
Fiber: 3g

LENTIL SOUP WITH VEGETABLES

Ingredients:

1 cup dried lentils
1 onion
2 carrots
2 celery stalks
4 cups vegetable broth
2 cloves garlic
1 teaspoon cumin
1 teaspoon paprika
Salt and pepper to taste

Instructions:

Rinse and drain the lentils.
Chop the onion, carrots, and celery.
In a large pot, sauté the onion, carrots, and celery in olive oil until softened.
Add garlic, cumin, paprika, and lentils to the pot and stir.
Add vegetable broth and bring to a boil.
Reduce heat to low and simmer for 30-40 minutes or until lentils are tender.
Season with salt and pepper to taste.

Nutrition information per serving:

Calories: 221
Protein: 16g
Fat: 1g
Carbohydrates: 39g
Fiber: 16g

GRILLED STEAK WITH ROASTED SWEET POTATOES

Ingredients:

4 sirloin steaks
4 sweet potatoes
1 tablespoon olive oil

Salt and pepper to taste

Instructions:

Preheat grill to medium-high heat.
Season the steaks with salt and pepper.
Peel and dice the sweet potatoes into bite-sized pieces.
Toss the sweet potatoes with olive oil, salt, and pepper.
Grill the steaks for 4-5 minutes per side or until cooked to your liking.
Roast the sweet potatoes in the oven at 400°F (200°C) for 20-25 minutes or until tender.

Nutrition information per serving:

Calories: 433
Protein: 42g
Fat: 16g
Carbohydrates: 30g
Fiber: 5g

GRILLED SALMON WITH LEMON AND HERBS

Ingredients:

4 salmon fillets

2 tbsp. olive oil
1 lemon, sliced
2 cloves garlic, minced
1 tbsp. fresh thyme
Salt and pepper

Instructions:

Preheat grill to medium-high heat.
In a small bowl, mix together olive oil, garlic, thyme, salt, and pepper.
Brush salmon fillets with the mixture on both sides.
Place the lemon slices on top of the fillets.
Grill for 5-7 minutes on each side, or until cooked through.
Serve hot.

Nutrition Information (per serving):

Calories: 307
Protein: 34g
Fat: 18g
Carbs: 2g

CHICKEN FAJITAS

Ingredients:

2 boneless, skinless chicken breasts, sliced

1 green bell pepper, sliced
1 red bell pepper, sliced
1 onion, sliced
1 tbsp. olive oil
1 tsp. chili powder
1 tsp. cumin
Salt and pepper
Flour tortillas

Instructions:

Heat olive oil in a large skillet over medium-high heat.
Add chicken, peppers, onion, chili powder, cumin, salt, and pepper.
Cook for 8-10 minutes, or until chicken is cooked through and vegetables are tender.
Serve with warm flour tortillas.

Nutrition Information (per serving):

Calories: 321
Protein: 28g
Fat: 10g
Carbs: 29g

BEEF STIR-FRY

Ingredients:

1 lb. beef sirloin, sliced
1 onion, sliced
2 bell peppers, sliced
1 cup broccoli florets
2 tbsp. vegetable oil
2 cloves garlic, minced
Salt and pepper

Instructions:

Heat vegetable oil in a large skillet over high heat.
Add beef and garlic and cook for 3-4 minutes, or until browned.
Add onion, peppers, and broccoli and cook for 5-7 minutes, or until vegetables are tender.
Season with salt and pepper.
Serve hot.

Nutrition Information (Per Serving):

Calories: 404
Protein: 31g
Fat: 25g
Carbs: 13g

TURKEY CHILI

Ingredients:

1 lb. ground turkey
1 onion, chopped
2 cloves garlic, minced
1 can kidney beans, drained and rinsed
1 can diced tomatoes
1 tbsp. chili powder
1 tsp. cumin
Salt and pepper

Instructions:

In a large pot, cook ground turkey over medium heat until browned.
Add onion and garlic and cook until onion is translucent.
Add kidney beans, tomatoes, chili powder, cumin, salt, and pepper.
Bring to a boil, then reduce heat and simmer for 20-30 minutes.
Serve hot.

Nutrition Information (Per Serving):

Calories: 294
Protein: 25g
Fat: 6g
Carbs: 33g

GRILLED CHICKEN WITH AVOCADO SALSA

Ingredients:

4 boneless, skinless chicken breasts
2 tbsp. olive oil
2 avocados, diced
1 tomato, diced
1/4 cup red onion, diced
2 tbsp. fresh cilantro, chopped
1 lime, juiced
Salt and pepper

Instructions:

Preheat grill to medium-high heat.
Brush chicken breasts with olive oil and season with salt and pepper.
Grill for 5-7 minutes on each side, or until cooked through.
In a small bowl, mix together diced avocado, tomato, red onion, cilantro, lime juice, salt, and pepper.
Serve grilled chicken with avocado salsa on top.

Nutrition Information (per serving):

Calories: 373
Protein: 31g

Fat: 23g
Carbs: 15g

TUNA SALAD LETTUCE WRAPS

Ingredients:

2 cans tuna, drained
1/2 cup celery, diced
1/4 cup red onion, diced
1/4 cup mayonnaise
1 tbsp. Dijon mustard
Salt and pepper
Lettuce leaves

Instructions:

In a medium bowl, mix together tuna, celery, red onion, mayonnaise, Dijon mustard, salt, and pepper.
Spoon the tuna salad onto lettuce leaves.
Roll up and serve.

Nutrition Information (Per Serving):

Calories: 203
Protein: 24g
Fat: 9g
Carbs: 4g

BAKED COD WITH LEMON AND GARLIC

Ingredients:

4 cod fillets
2 tbsp. olive oil
2 cloves garlic, minced
1 lemon, juiced
Salt and pepper

Instructions:

Preheat oven to 375°F.
Brush cod fillets with olive oil and place in a baking
dish.
Sprinkle minced garlic on top of the fillets.
Squeeze lemon juice over the fillets.
Season with salt and pepper.
Bake for 12-15 minutes, or until cooked through.
Serve hot.

Nutrition Information (per serving):

Calories: 184
Protein: 31g
Fat: 6g
Carbs: 2g

QUINOA AND BLACK BEAN BOWL

Ingredients:

1 cup quinoa, cooked
1 can black beans, drained and rinsed
1 red bell pepper, chopped
1/4 cup red onion, chopped
2 tbsp. fresh cilantro, chopped
1 lime, juiced
Salt and pepper

Instructions:

In a large bowl, mix together cooked quinoa, black beans, red bell pepper, red onion, cilantro, lime juice, salt, and pepper.
Serve hot or cold.

Nutrition Information (per serving):

Calories: 313
Protein: 14g
Fat: 4g
Carbs: 56g

GRILLED STEAK WITH CHIMICHURRI SAUCE

Ingredients:

4 ribeye steaks
2 tbsp. olive oil
1/2 cup fresh parsley, chopped
1/4 cup fresh cilantro, chopped
3 cloves garlic, minced
1/4 cup red wine vinegar
1/2 cup olive oil
Salt and pepper

Instructions:

Preheat grill to medium-high heat.
Brush steaks with olive oil and season with salt and pepper.
Grill for 5-7 minutes on each side, or until desired doneness
In a small bowl, mix together chopped parsley, cilantro, minced garlic, red wine vinegar, olive oil, salt, and pepper.
Serve grilled steak with chimichurri sauce on top.

Nutrition Information (per serving):

Calories: 455
Protein: 33g
Fat: 34g
Carbs: 2g

LENTIL AND VEGETABLE STIR FRY

Ingredients:

1 cup brown lentils, cooked
1 bell pepper, sliced
1 zucchini, sliced
1 carrot, sliced
1/4 cup red onion, chopped
2 tbsp. soy sauce
2 tbsp. hoisin sauce
1 tbsp. sesame oil
Salt and pepper

Instructions:

In a large skillet, heat sesame oil over medium-high heat.
Add sliced bell pepper, zucchini, carrot, and red onion.
Stir fry for 5-7 minutes, or until vegetables are cooked through.
Add cooked lentils to the skillet and stir to combine.
Add soy sauce and hoisin sauce to the skillet and stir to coat vegetables and lentils.
Season with salt and pepper to taste.
Serve hot.

Nutrition Information (per serving):

Calories: 311
Protein: 16g
Fat: 7g
Carbs: 47g

BEEF AND BROCCOLI STIR FRY

Ingredients:

1 lb. flank steak, sliced
1 broccoli crown, chopped
1 red bell pepper, sliced
2 cloves garlic, minced
2 tbsp. soy sauce
1 tbsp. honey
1 tbsp. cornstarch
1 tbsp. sesame oil
Salt and pepper

Instructions:

In a small bowl, mix together soy sauce, honey, and cornstarch.
In a large skillet, heat sesame oil over medium-high heat.
Add sliced flank steak to the skillet and stir fry for 3-5 minutes, or until cooked through.

Add chopped broccoli and sliced red bell pepper to the skillet and stir fry for an additional 3-5 minutes, or until vegetables are cooked through.
Add minced garlic to the skillet and stir fry for 1 minute, or until fragrant.
Pour soy sauce mixture into the skillet and stir to coat beef and vegetables.
Season with salt and pepper to taste.
Serve hot.

Nutrition Information (per serving):

Calories: 364
Protein: 33g
Fat: 15g
Carbs: 23g

CHICKEN AND VEGETABLE KABOBS

Ingredients:

4 boneless, skinless chicken breasts, cubed
1 red bell pepper, cubed
1 green bell pepper, cubed
1 red onion, cubed
2 tbsp. olive oil
2 tbsp. balsamic vinegar
Salt and pepper

Instructions:

Preheat grill to medium-high heat.
Thread chicken, red bell pepper, green bell pepper, and red onion onto skewers.
Brush kabobs with olive oil and balsamic vinegar.
Season with salt and pepper.
Grill for 10-12 minutes, or until chicken is cooked through.
Serve hot.

Nutrition Information (per serving):

Calories: 292
Protein: 33g
Fat: 12g
Carbs: 12g

VEGETARIAN AND NON-VEGETARIAN OPTIONS

VEGETARIAN OPTIONS:

GRILLED PORTOBELLO MUSHROOM BURGER

Ingredients:

4 large Portobello mushrooms

4 burger buns
1 sliced tomato
1 sliced onion
Lettuce leaves
4 slices of cheese (optional)

Instructions:

Clean and remove the stems from the Portobello mushrooms.
Preheat the grill or a grill pan over medium heat.
Brush the mushrooms with olive oil and season with salt and pepper.
Grill the mushrooms for 4-5 minutes on each side.
Toast the burger buns.
Assemble the burger by placing a grilled mushroom on the bottom bun, followed by lettuce, tomato, onion, and cheese (if using).
Top with the remaining bun.

Nutritional Information (per serving):

Calories: 330
Protein: 15g
Fat: 11g
Carbohydrates: 45g
Fiber: 6g
Sugar: 10g

VEGETARIAN CHILI

Ingredients:

1 can of black beans, drained and rinsed
1 can of kidney beans, drained and rinsed
1 can of corn, drained
1 can of diced tomatoes
1 diced onion
1 diced red bell pepper
1 tablespoon of olive oil
1 tablespoon of chili powder
1 teaspoon of ground cumin
Salt and pepper to taste

Instructions:

Heat the olive oil in a large pot over medium heat.
Add the diced onion and red bell pepper and sauté for 5-7 minutes.
Add the chili powder, ground cumin, salt, and pepper, and stir.
Add the black beans, kidney beans, corn, and diced tomatoes.
Stir well and bring to a boil.
Reduce the heat to low and simmer for 20-25 minutes.
Serve hot.

Nutritional Information (per serving):

Calories: 235
Protein: 11g
Fat: 5g
Carbohydrates: 40g
Fiber: 10g
Sugar: 7g

CAPRESE SALAD

Ingredients:

2 large tomatoes, sliced
8 ounces of fresh mozzarella, sliced
¼ cup of fresh basil leaves
1 tablespoon of balsamic vinegar
1 tablespoon of olive oil
Salt and pepper to taste

Instructions:

Arrange the sliced tomatoes and fresh mozzarella on a plate.
Sprinkle the basil leaves over the top.
Drizzle with balsamic vinegar and olive oil.
Season with salt and pepper to taste.
Serve immediately.

Nutritional Information (per serving):

Calories: 290
Protein: 19g
Fat: 21g
Carbohydrates: 9g
Fiber: 2g
Sugar: 5g

VEGETABLE STIR-FRY

Ingredients:

1 tablespoon of olive oil
1 diced onion
1 diced red bell pepper
1 diced yellow bell pepper
2 sliced carrots
1 sliced zucchini
1 tablespoon of soy sauce
Salt and pepper to taste

Instructions:

Heat the olive oil in a large skillet or wok over medium-high heat.
Add the diced onion and sauté for 2-3 minutes.
Add the red and yellow bell peppers and sauté for 2-3 minutes.

Add the sliced carrots and sauté for 2-3 minutes.
Add the sliced zucchini and sauté for 2-3 minutes.
Drizzle with soy sauce and season with salt and pepper to taste.
Serve hot.

Nutritional Information (per serving):

Calories: 120
Protein: 3g
Fat: 6g
Carbohydrates: 14g
Fiber: 4g
Sugar: 8g

NON-VEGETARIAN OPTIONS:

GRILLED CHICKEN SALAD

Ingredients:

8 ounces of grilled chicken breast, sliced
2 cups of mixed greens
1 diced tomato
1 diced cucumber
1 diced red onion
2 tablespoons of balsamic vinaigrette

Instructions:

Grill the chicken breast until fully cooked.

Assemble the salad by placing mixed greens on a plate.

Add the sliced chicken, diced tomato, cucumber, and red onion.

Drizzle with balsamic vinaigrette.

Serve immediately.

Nutritional Information (per serving):

Calories: 280
Protein: 35g
Fat: 10g
Carbohydrates: 13g
Fiber: 4g
Sugar: 7g

BAKED SALMON WITH LEMON AND DILL

Ingredients:

4 salmon fillets
1 sliced lemon
2 tablespoons of chopped fresh dill
1 tablespoon of olive oil
Salt and pepper to taste

Instructions:

Preheat the oven to 375°F.
Line a baking sheet with parchment paper.
Brush the salmon fillets with olive oil and season with salt and pepper.
Place the salmon fillets on the prepared baking sheet.
Top each fillet with sliced lemon and chopped dill.
Bake for 12-15 minutes, or until the salmon is cooked through.
Serve hot.

Nutritional Information (per serving):

Calories: 330
Protein: 36g
Fat: 18g
Carbohydrates: 2g
Fiber: 0g
Sugar: 0g

BEEF STIR-FRY

Ingredients:

1 pound of beef sirloin, thinly sliced
1 tablespoon of cornstarch
2 tablespoons of soy sauce
1 tablespoon of vegetable oil

1 sliced onion
1 sliced red bell pepper
1 sliced green bell pepper
Salt and pepper to taste

Instructions:

In a small bowl, mix the cornstarch and soy sauce.
Add the sliced beef to the bowl and toss to coat.
Heat the vegetable oil in a large skillet or wok over
high heat.
Add the sliced onion and sauté for 2-3 minutes.
Add the sliced red and green bell peppers and sauté
for 2-3 minutes.
Add the beef and cook for 2-3 minutes.
Season with salt and pepper to taste.
Serve hot.

Nutritional Information (per serving):

Calories: 350
Protein: 30g
Fat: 22g
Carbohydrates: 8g
Fiber: 2g
Sugar: 4g

GRILLED SHRIMP SKEWERS

Ingredients:

1 pound of large shrimp, peeled and deveined
1 sliced bell pepper
1 sliced red onion
1 tablespoon of olive oil
Salt and pepper to taste

Instructions:

Preheat the grill to medium-high heat.
Thread the shrimp, bell pepper, and red onion onto skewers.
Brush the skewers with olive oil and season with salt and pepper.
Grill the skewers for 2-3 minutes per side, or until the shrimp are cooked through.
Serve hot.

Nutritional Information (per serving):

Calories: 180
Protein: 22g
Fat: 7g
Carbohydrates: 7g
Fiber: 2g
Sugar: 4g

PORK CHOPS WITH APPLE COMPOTE

Ingredients:

4 bone-in pork chops
2 sliced apples
2 tablespoons of butter
2 tablespoons of brown sugar
1 tablespoon of apple cider vinegar
1 teaspoon of cinnamon
Salt and pepper to taste

Instructions:

Preheat the oven to 375°F.
Season the pork chops with salt and pepper.
Heat a large skillet over medium-high heat.
Add the pork chops to the skillet and cook for 2-3 minutes per side, or until browned.
Transfer the pork chops to a baking dish.
In the same skillet, melt the butter over medium heat.
Add the sliced apples, brown sugar, apple cider vinegar, cinnamon, salt, and pepper.
Cook the apple mixture for 2-3 minutes, or until the apples are tender.
Pour the apple mixture over the pork chops in the baking dish.
Bake for 20-25 minutes, or until the pork chops are cooked through.

Serve hot.

Nutritional Information (per serving):

Calories: 400
Protein: 31g
Fat: 20g
Carbohydrates: 24g
Fiber: 4g
Sugar: 18g

BEEF AND BROCCOLI STIR-FRY

Ingredients:

1 pound of beef sirloin, thinly sliced
2 cups of broccoli florets
1 sliced onion
1 tablespoon of cornstarch
2 tablespoons of soy sauce
1 tablespoon of vegetable oil
Salt and pepper to taste

Instructions:

In a small bowl, mix the cornstarch and soy sauce.
Add the sliced beef to the bowl and toss to coat.
Heat the vegetable oil in a large skillet or wok over
high heat.

Add the sliced onion and sauté for 2-3 minutes.
Add the broccoli florets and sauté for 2-3 minutes.
Add the beef and cook for 2-3 minutes.
Season with salt and pepper to taste.
Serve hot.

Nutritional Information (per serving):

Calories: 300
Protein: 30g
Fat: 12g
Carbohydrates: 16g
Fiber: 4g
Sugar: 6g

CHAPTER 6

HIGH-CALORIE SNACK RECIPES

Here are three high-calorie snack recipes that are perfect for men, along with instructions and nutritional information:

PEANUT BUTTER AND BANANA SMOOTHIE

Ingredients:

1 banana
1/2 cup of milk
1/2 cup of plain Greek yogurt
1 tablespoon of peanut butter
1 tablespoon of honey
1/2 teaspoon of vanilla extract
Ice cubes (optional)

Instructions:

Peel the banana and chop it into small pieces.
Add the banana, milk, Greek yogurt, peanut butter, honey, and vanilla extract to a blender.
Blend the ingredients until smooth. If the smoothie is too thick, you can add a few ice cubes and blend again.

Pour the smoothie into a glass and enjoy!

Nutritional Information:

Calories: 400
Protein: 23g
Carbohydrates: 51g
Fat: 14g
Fiber: 4g

AVOCADO TOAST WITH EGG

Ingredients:

2 slices of whole grain bread
1 ripe avocado
2 eggs
Salt and pepper
Olive oil

Instructions:

Toast the bread slices in a toaster.
Cut the avocado in half and remove the pit. Scoop out the flesh and mash it with a fork in a small bowl.
Heat a small amount of olive oil in a nonstick pan over medium heat.

Crack the eggs into the pan and cook until the whites are set and the yolks are runny. Season with salt and pepper to taste.
Spread the mashed avocado on each slice of toast.
Top each slice with one fried egg.
Serve immediately.

Nutritional Information:

Calories: 600
Protein: 24g
Carbohydrates: 44g
Fat: 40g
Fiber: 16g

TRAIL MIX

Ingredients:

1/2 cup of almonds
1/2 cup of cashews
1/2 cup of peanuts
1/2 cup of dried cranberries
1/2 cup of dark chocolate chips

Instructions:

Add all the ingredients to a bowl.
Mix well.

Divide the trail mix into individual servings and store in small ziplock bags.

Nutritional Information:

Calories: 500
Protein: 15g
Carbohydrates: 30g
Fat: 38g
Fiber: 7g

IMPORTANCE OF SNACKING FOR WEIGHT GAIN

Snacking can be an important part of a weight gain strategy for some people. When trying to gain weight, it's important to consume more calories than you burn, and snacking can help you achieve this goal by increasing your overall calorie intake.

Snacks can also help you maintain your energy levels throughout the day, especially if you have a fast metabolism or a physically demanding job. Eating small, frequent meals can prevent dips in blood sugar levels, which can cause fatigue and cravings for unhealthy foods.

However, it's important to choose healthy, high-calorie snacks that will fuel your body and provide the nutrients you need. Examples include nuts and seeds, dried fruits, avocados, cheese, whole-grain crackers, and protein bars.

It's also important to keep portion sizes in mind and not overdo it on snacking. Aim for snacks that are around 200-300 calories each, and try to eat them in between meals rather than as a replacement for them.

Overall, snacking can be a useful tool for weight gain, but it's important to make healthy choices and practice moderation.

HIGH-CALORIE SNACK RECIPE IDEAS

CHOCOLATE PEANUT BUTTER ENERGY BALLS

Ingredients:

1 cup rolled oats
1/2 cup creamy peanut butter
1/4 cup honey
1/4 cup chocolate chips
1/4 cup chopped nuts (optional)

Instructions:

In a mixing bowl, combine oats, peanut butter, and honey.

Mix in chocolate chips and nuts, if using.

Roll the mixture into 1-inch balls and place on a baking sheet lined with parchment paper.

Refrigerate for at least 30 minutes before serving.

Nutritional Information (per serving, based on 12 servings):

Calories: 159
Fat: 8g
Protein: 5g
Carbs: 19g
Fiber: 2g
Sugar: 10g

AVOCADO TOAST WITH FRIED EGG

Ingredients:

2 slices whole grain bread
1 ripe avocado
2 eggs
Salt and pepper
Olive oil

Instructions:

Toast the bread and set aside.

Mash the avocado and spread it evenly on the toasted bread.

Heat a small nonstick pan over medium-high heat and add a drizzle of olive oil.

Crack the eggs into the pan and cook to your desired level of doneness.

Season with salt and pepper, and place the fried egg on top of the avocado toast.

Nutritional Information (per serving):

Calories: 484
Fat: 31g
Protein: 16g
Carbs: 38g
Fiber: 13g
Sugar: 3g

NUTELLA AND BANANA CREPES

Ingredients:

2 crepes (store-bought or homemade)
2 tbsp Nutella
1 ripe banana, sliced
Whipped cream (optional)

Instructions:

Warm the crepes in the microwave for 10 seconds, if needed.
Spread Nutella evenly over each crepe.
Add sliced bananas on top of the Nutella.
Roll up the crepes and top with whipped cream, if desired.

Nutritional Information (per serving):

Calories: 455
Fat: 20g
Protein: 9g
Carbs: 63g
Fiber: 5g
Sugar: 32g

HOMEMADE TRAIL MIX

Ingredients:

1 cup roasted almonds
1 cup dried cranberries
1 cup dark chocolate chips
1 cup banana chips

Instructions:

Mix all ingredients together in a large bowl.

Store in an airtight container for up to 1 week.

Nutritional Information (per serving, based on 8 servings):

Calories: 383
Fat: 23g
Protein: 6g
Carbs: 43g
Fiber: 6g
Sugar: 29g

LOADED SWEET POTATO FRIES

Ingredients:

2 medium sweet potatoes
1 tbsp olive oil
1/4 cup shredded cheddar cheese
2 tbsp cooked bacon bits
2 tbsp chopped green onions
Salt and pepper

Instructions:

Preheat oven to 425°F (218°C).
Slice sweet potatoes into thin fries.
Toss with olive oil, salt, and pepper.

Spread fries in a single layer on a baking sheet lined with parchment paper.
Bake for 20-25 minutes, until crispy.
Top with shredded cheese, bacon bits, and green onions.

Nutritional Information (per serving):

Calories: 438
Fat: 19g
Protein: 12g
Carbs: 58g
Fiber: 8g
Sugar: 16g

PEANUT BUTTER BANANA SMOOTHIE

Ingredients:

1 banana
1/2 cup creamy peanut butter
1 cup milk
1/4 cup honey
1 tsp vanilla extract
1 cup ice

Instructions:

Add all ingredients to a blender.

Blend until smooth.
Pour into a glass and serve immediately.

Nutritional Information (per serving):

Calories: 569
Fat: 34g
Protein: 19g
Carbs: 53g
Fiber: 4g
Sugar: 44g

CHEESY BACON DIP

Ingredients:

8 oz cream cheese, softened
1/2 cup sour cream
1/2 cup shredded cheddar cheese
1/2 cup cooked bacon bits
2 tbsp chopped green onions

Instructions:

In a mixing bowl, combine cream cheese and sour
cream until smooth.
Mix in shredded cheddar cheese, bacon bits, and
green onions.

Serve with crackers, chips, or vegetables for dipping.

Nutritional Information (per serving, based on 8 servings):

Calories: 209
Fat: 19g
Protein: 7g
Carbs: 2g
Fiber: 0g
Sugar: 1g

LOADED NACHOS

Ingredients:

8 oz tortilla chips
1 cup shredded cheddar cheese
1/2 cup cooked ground beef
1/2 cup black beans
1/4 cup sliced jalapeños
1/4 cup chopped tomatoes
1/4 cup chopped green onions
Sour cream and guacamole for serving

Instructions:

Preheat oven to 375°F (190°C).

Arrange tortilla chips on a baking sheet lined with parchment paper.

Sprinkle shredded cheddar cheese over the tortilla chips.

Add cooked ground beef, black beans, jalapeños, tomatoes, and green onions.

Bake for 10-12 minutes, until cheese is melted and bubbly.

Serve with sour cream and guacamole.

Nutritional Information (per serving):

Calories: 809
Fat: 49g
Protein: 25g
Carbs: 66g
Fiber: 10g
Sugar: 4g

CHOCOLATE BANANA PROTEIN SHAKE

Ingredients:

1 banana
1 scoop chocolate protein powder
1 cup milk
1 tbsp peanut butter
1 cup ice

Instructions:

Add all ingredients to a blender.
Blend until smooth.
Pour into a glass and serve immediately.

Nutritional Information (per serving):

Calories: 484
Fat: 19g
Protein: 34g
Carbs: 49g
Fiber: 5g
Sugar: 29g

BAKED BRIE WITH HONEY AND ALMONDS

Ingredients:

1 wheel of brie cheese
1/4 cup honey
1/4 cup sliced almonds

Instructions:

Preheat oven to 350°F (177°C).
Place the brie cheese in a baking dish.
Drizzle honey over the brie.
Sprinkle sliced almonds on top.

Nutritional Information (per serving):

Calories: 433
Fat: 28g
Protein: 11g
Carbs: 34g
Fiber: 5g
Sugar: 20g

CHAPTER 7

HEALTHY FATS RECIPES

AVOCADO TOAST WITH SMOKED SALMON:

Ingredients:

1 slice of whole-grain bread
1/4 avocado
1 oz smoked salmon
1/4 lemon
Salt and pepper to taste

Instructions:

Toast the bread to your desired level of crispiness.
Mash the avocado in a small bowl and add salt and pepper to taste.
Spread the mashed avocado on the toast.
Place the smoked salmon on top of the avocado.
Squeeze the lemon juice over the salmon.
Enjoy!

Nutrition Information (per serving):

Calories: 235
Fat: 11g
Carbohydrates: 18g
Protein: 16g

ROASTED BRUSSELS SPROUTS WITH BACON:

Ingredients:

1 lb Brussels sprouts
2 slices of bacon
1 tbsp olive oil
Salt and pepper to taste

Instructions:

Preheat the oven to 400°F.
Wash the Brussels sprouts and cut off the ends.
Cut the bacon into small pieces.
In a large bowl, toss the Brussels sprouts with olive oil, salt, and pepper.
Add the bacon to the bowl and mix well.
Spread the Brussels sprouts and bacon mixture onto a baking sheet.
Roast in the oven for 25-30 minutes or until the Brussels sprouts are crispy.
Enjoy!

Nutrition Information (per serving):

Calories: 165
Fat: 10g
Carbohydrates: 12g
Protein: 9g

CHIA SEED PUDDING WITH ALMOND MILK:

Ingredients:

2 tbsp chia seeds
1 cup unsweetened almond milk
1/2 tsp vanilla extract
1/2 tsp cinnamon
1 tsp honey (optional)

Instructions:

In a bowl, mix the chia seeds, almond milk, vanilla extract, and cinnamon.
Stir well to make sure the chia seeds are evenly distributed.
Cover the bowl with plastic wrap and refrigerate for at least 2 hours or overnight.
If you want to sweeten the pudding, add honey to taste before serving.
Enjoy!

Nutrition Information (per serving):

Calories: 131
Fat: 8g
Carbohydrates: 13g
Protein: 4g

IMPORTANCE OF HEALTHY FATS IN WEIGHT GAIN DIET

When it comes to gaining weight, it's important to focus on consuming nutrient-dense foods that provide the body with the necessary nutrients to build muscle and support overall health. Healthy fats are an important part of a weight gain diet for several reasons:

They are calorie-dense: Healthy fats provide more calories per gram than protein or carbohydrates, making them an efficient way to increase calorie intake and promote weight gain.

They support hormone production: Hormones such as testosterone and estrogen are crucial for muscle growth and overall health. Healthy fats are essential for the production of these hormones.

They improve nutrient absorption: Many essential vitamins and minerals are fat-soluble, meaning they are better absorbed when consumed with healthy fats. This ensures that the body is able to absorb and utilize all the nutrients from the foods consumed.

They provide energy: Healthy fats are an excellent source of energy for the body. Consuming them can help prevent fatigue and provide the energy needed for intense workouts.

Examples of healthy fats that can be included in a weight gain diet include avocados, nuts and seeds, olive oil, coconut oil, fatty fish (such as salmon), and full-fat dairy products. It's important to note that while healthy fats are beneficial for weight gain, they should still be consumed in moderation as excess calorie intake can lead to unwanted weight gain.

HEALTHY FATS RECIPE IDEAS

AVOCADO TOAST

Ingredients:

1 slice whole wheat bread
1/2 avocado
Salt and pepper to taste
Optional toppings: sliced tomato, red onion, microgreens, feta cheese

Instructions:

Toast the bread until golden brown.
While the bread is toasting, mash the avocado in a small bowl with salt and pepper.
Spread the mashed avocado on the toast.
Add any desired toppings.
Enjoy!

Nutrition Information (per serving):

Calories: 213
Fat: 13g
Carbohydrates: 22g
Protein: 5g

ROASTED BRUSSELS SPROUTS WITH BACON AND PECANS

Ingredients:

1 lb. Brussels sprouts, trimmed and halved
4 slices bacon, chopped
1/2 cup pecans, chopped
Salt and pepper to taste
Olive oil

Instructions:

Preheat oven to 400°F.

In a large bowl, toss the Brussels sprouts with enough olive oil to coat them.

Spread the Brussels sprouts on a baking sheet.

Roast for 20-25 minutes, or until the sprouts are tender and browned.

While the Brussels sprouts are roasting, cook the bacon in a large skillet until crisp.

Add the chopped pecans to the skillet and cook until toasted.

Toss the roasted Brussels sprouts with the bacon and pecans.

Season with salt and pepper to taste.

Enjoy!

Nutrition Information (per serving):

Calories: 214
Fat: 16g
Carbohydrates: 12g
Protein: 8g

SALMON AND AVOCADO SALAD

Ingredients:

2 cups mixed greens
1/2 avocado, diced

1/2 cup cherry tomatoes, halved
1/4 red onion, thinly sliced
4 oz. cooked salmon
1 tbsp. olive oil
1 tbsp. lemon juice
Salt and pepper to taste

Instructions :

In a large bowl, toss the mixed greens, avocado, cherry tomatoes, and red onion.
Flake the cooked salmon and add it to the bowl.
In a small bowl, whisk together the olive oil, lemon juice, salt, and pepper.
Drizzle the dressing over the salad and toss to combine.
Enjoy!

Nutrition Information (per serving):

Calories: 318
Fat: 23g
Carbohydrates: 12g
Protein: 18g

ALMOND BUTTER BANANA SMOOTHIE

Ingredients:

1 banana
1 tbsp. almond butter
1/2 cup almond milk
1/4 tsp. cinnamon
1/2 tsp. honey
1/2 cup ice cubes

Instructions:

Add all ingredients to a blender and blend until smooth.
Enjoy!

Nutrition Information (per serving):

Calories: 231
Fat: 12g
Carbohydrates: 28g
Protein: 5g

DARK CHOCOLATE AVOCADO MOUSSE

Ingredients:

2 ripe avocados
1/4 cup unsweetened cocoa powder
1/4 cup maple syrup
1/4 cup almond milk
1 tsp. vanilla extract

Instructions:

Add all ingredients to a blender or food processor and blend until smooth.
Divide the mixture into 4 small bowls or ramekins.
Refrigerate for at least 30 minutes, or until set.
Enjoy!

Nutrition Information (per serving):

Calories: 220
Fat: 15g
Carbohydrates: 24g
Protein: 3g

QUINOA AND AVOCADO SALAD

Ingredients:

1 cup cooked quinoa
1 avocado, diced
1/2 cup cherry tomatoes, halved
1/4 cup red onion, diced
1/4 cup cilantro, chopped
1 tbsp. olive oil
1 tbsp. lime juice
Salt and pepper to taste

Instructions:

In a large bowl, combine the quinoa, avocado, cherry tomatoes, red onion, and cilantro.
In a small bowl, whisk together the olive oil, lime juice, salt, and pepper.
Drizzle the dressing over the salad and toss to combine.
Enjoy!

Nutrition Information (per serving):

Calories: 333
Fat: 18g
Carbohydrates: 36g
Protein: 8g

CHIA SEED PUDDING

Ingredients:

1/4 cup chia seeds
1 cup almond milk
1 tbsp. maple syrup
1/4 tsp. vanilla extract
Optional toppings: sliced banana, berries, nuts

Instructions:

In a bowl, whisk together the chia seeds, almond milk, maple syrup, and vanilla extract.
Refrigerate for at least 2 hours, or until the mixture has thickened into a pudding-like consistency.
Top with desired toppings.
Enjoy!

Nutrition Information (per serving):

Calories: 189
Fat: 9g
Carbohydrates: 23g
Protein: 6g

ROASTED SWEET POTATOES WITH TAHINI SAUCE

Ingredients:

2 large sweet potatoes, peeled and cubed
2 tbsp. olive oil
Salt and pepper to taste
1/4 cup tahini
2 tbsp. lemon juice
2 tbsp. water
1 garlic clove, minced
Optional toppings: chopped parsley, pomegranate seeds

Instructions:

Preheat oven to 400°F.
In a large bowl, toss the sweet potatoes with olive oil, salt, and pepper.
Spread the sweet potatoes on a baking sheet.
Roast for 25-30 minutes, or until tender and browned.
While the sweet potatoes are roasting, prepare the tahini sauce by whisking together the tahini, lemon juice, water, garlic, and salt in a small bowl.
Drizzle the tahini sauce over the roasted sweet potatoes.
Top with desired toppings.
Enjoy!

Nutrition Information (per serving):

Calories: 316
Fat: 19g
Carbohydrates: 33g
Protein: 6g

BAKED SALMON WITH AVOCADO SALSA

Ingredients:

4 salmon fillets
1 avocado, diced

1/2 cup cherry tomatoes, halved
1/4 cup red onion, diced
1/4 cup cilantro, chopped
1 lime, juiced
1 tbsp. olive oil
Salt and pepper to taste

Instructions:

Preheat oven to 400°F.
Season the salmon fillets with salt and pepper.
Place the salmon fillets on a baking sheet and bake for 12-15 minutes, or until cooked through.
In a bowl, combine the avocado, cherry tomatoes, red onion, cilantro, lime juice, olive oil, salt, and pepper.
Serve the salmon fillets with the avocado salsa on top.
Enjoy!

Nutrition Information (per serving):

Calories: 422
Fat: 27g
Carbohydrates: 11g
Protein: 34g

ALMOND BUTTER AND BANANA SMOOTHIE

Ingredients:

1 banana, frozen
1 cup almond milk
2 tbsp. almond butter
1 tsp. honey
1/4 tsp. cinnamon

Instructions:

Add all ingredients to a blender and blend until smooth.
Pour into a glass and serve immediately.
Enjoy!

Nutrition Information (per serving):

Calories: 307
Fat: 17g
Carbohydrates: 33g
Protein: 8g

AVOCADO TOAST WITH POACHED EGG

Ingredients:

2 slices of whole grain bread
1 avocado, mashed
2 eggs

1 tbsp. white vinegar
Salt and pepper to taste

Instructions:

Toast the bread slices.
Spread the mashed avocado evenly over the toast.
Fill a medium saucepan with water and bring to a boil.
Add the white vinegar to the water.
Crack each egg into a separate ramekin or small bowl.
Reduce the heat of the water to a simmer and stir the water to create a vortex.
Carefully drop each egg into the center of the vortex.
Cook the eggs for 3-4 minutes, or until the whites are set but the yolks are still runny.
Remove the eggs from the water with a slotted spoon and place on top of the avocado toast.
Season with salt and pepper.
Enjoy!

Nutrition Information (per serving):

Calories: 390
Fat: 25g
Carbohydrates: 28g
Protein: 17g

ROASTED CAULIFLOWER WITH TAHINI DRESSING

Ingredients:

1 head cauliflower, chopped into florets
2 tbsp. olive oil
Salt and pepper to taste
1/4 cup tahini
1/4 cup lemon juice
1 garlic clove, minced
2 tbsp. water

Instructions:

Preheat oven to 425°F.
In a large bowl, toss the cauliflower florets with olive oil, salt, and pepper.
Spread the cauliflower on a baking sheet and roast for 20-25 minutes, or until golden brown and tender.
In a small bowl, whisk together the tahini, lemon juice, garlic, and water until smooth.
Drizzle the tahini dressing over the roasted cauliflower.
Serve immediately.
Enjoy!

Nutrition Information (per serving):

Calories: 222
Fat: 17g
Carbohydrates: 13g
Protein: 6g

CHOCOLATE CHIA SEED PUDDING

Ingredients:

1/4 cup chia seeds
1 cup unsweetened almond milk
2 tbsp. cocoa powder
1 tbsp. honey
1/4 tsp. vanilla extract

Instructions:

In a bowl, whisk together the chia seeds, almond milk, cocoa powder, honey, and vanilla extract.
Cover and refrigerate overnight, or for at least 2 hours.
Stir the pudding before serving.
Enjoy!

Nutrition Information (per serving):

Calories: 219

Fat: 13g
Carbohydrates: 21g
Protein: 8g

GRILLED SHRIMP WITH MANGO SALSA

Ingredients:

1 lb. shrimp, peeled and deveined
1 tbsp. olive oil
Salt and pepper to taste
1 mango, diced
1/2 red onion, diced
1 jalapeño pepper, seeded and diced
1/4 cup cilantro, chopped
1 lime, juiced

Instructions:

Preheat grill to medium-high heat.
Toss the shrimp with olive oil, salt, and pepper.
Grill the shrimp for 2-3 minutes per side, or until cooked through.
In a bowl, combine the mango, red onion, jalapeño pepper, cilantro, lime juice, salt, and pepper.
Serve the grilled shrimp with the mango salsa on top.
Enjoy!

Nutrition Information (per serving):

Calories: 227
Fat: 8g
Carbohydrates: 14g
Protein: 25g

SPINACH SALAD WITH STRAWBERRIES AND WALNUTS

Ingredients:

4 cups baby spinach
1 cup strawberries, sliced
1/4 cup chopped walnuts
1/4 cup crumbled feta cheese
1 tbsp. olive oil
1 tbsp. balsamic vinegar
Salt and pepper to taste

Instructions:

In a large bowl, toss the spinach, strawberries, walnuts, and feta cheese.
In a small bowl, whisk together the olive oil, balsamic vinegar, salt, and pepper.
Drizzle the dressing over the salad and toss to coat.
Serve immediately.
Enjoy!

Nutrition Information (per serving):

Calories: 205
Fat: 15g
Carbohydrates: 12g

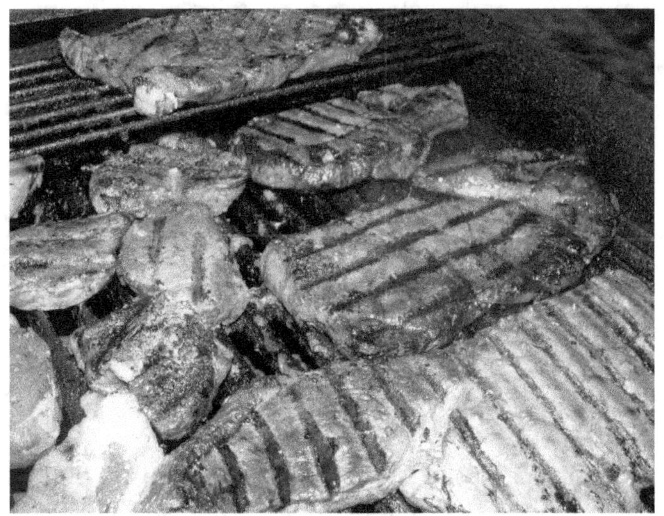

CHAPTER 8

SMOOTHIES AND SHAKES FOR WEIGHT GAIN

If you're looking to gain weight in a healthy way, smoothies and shakes can be a great addition to your diet. Here are some tips and recipes for making weight-gain smoothies and shakes:

Choose nutrient-dense ingredients: When making a weight-gain smoothie or shake, focus on using ingredients that are high in calories and nutrients. Good options include nut butters, avocados, full-fat dairy products, coconut oil, and fruits like bananas and mangos.

Use protein powder: Adding a scoop of protein powder to your smoothie or shake can help you meet your protein needs and support muscle growth. Look for a high-quality protein powder that contains at least 20 grams of protein per serving.

Add healthy fats: Healthy fats are an important part of a weight-gain diet, as they are calorie-dense and provide essential nutrients. Good options for adding healthy fats to your smoothie or shake include nuts, seeds, nut butters, avocado, and coconut oil.

Experiment with flavors: Smoothies and shakes can be customized to your taste preferences. Try different flavor combinations to keep things interesting and prevent boredom. Some ideas include chocolate and peanut butter, vanilla and almond, or berry and coconut.

Here are recipes for weight-gain smoothies and shakes:

CHOCOLATE PEANUT BUTTER SHAKE

1 cup whole milk
1 banana
1 scoop chocolate protein powder
2 tablespoons peanut butter
1 tablespoon honey
1/4 teaspoon vanilla extract

Blend all ingredients in a blender until smooth. Serve immediately.

MANGO COCONUT SMOOTHIE

1 cup coconut milk
1 cup frozen mango chunks
1 scoop vanilla protein powder
1 tablespoon coconut oil

1 teaspoon honey

Blend all ingredients in a blender until smooth. Serve immediately.

BERRY NUT SMOOTHIE

1 cup almond milk
1 cup frozen mixed berries
1 scoop vanilla protein powder
2 tablespoons almond butter
1 teaspoon honey

Blend all ingredients in a blender until smooth. Serve immediately.

HOW SMOOTHIES AND SHAKES CAN HELP IN WEIGHT GAIN

Smoothies and shakes can be effective tools for weight gain when used as part of a well-planned diet and exercise regimen. Here are a few ways they can help:

Convenient and calorie-dense: Smoothies and shakes are easy to make and can be packed with high-calorie ingredients like fruits, nuts, seeds, and nut butter. By blending these ingredients together, you can create a calorie-dense beverage that is easy to consume on the go.

Nutrient-rich: Smoothies and shakes can also be a good source of vitamins, minerals, and other nutrients that are important for overall health. By including ingredients like leafy greens, berries, and other whole foods, you can create a nutrient-rich drink that supports weight gain and good health.

Promote muscle growth: Protein is an essential nutrient for building muscle, and many smoothie and shake recipes include protein powder or other high-protein ingredients like Greek yogurt or cottage cheese. By consuming protein-rich smoothies and shakes after a workout or as a snack throughout the day, you can support muscle growth and repair.

It's important to note that simply drinking smoothies and shakes alone won't necessarily lead to weight gain. To see results, you'll need to consume these beverages as part of a balanced diet that includes plenty of whole foods and regular exercise. Additionally, it's important to choose smoothie and shake recipes that fit your dietary needs and preferences, and to monitor your calorie intake to ensure you're consuming enough to support weight gain.

RECIPES IDEAS FOR HIGH-CALORIE SMOOTHIES AND SHAKES

Here are some additional high-calorie smoothie and shake recipes

PEANUT BUTTER BANANA SHAKE

Ingredients:

1 banana
2 tbsp peanut butter
1 cup milk
1 scoop vanilla protein powder (optional)
1 tsp honey

Instructions:

Combine all ingredients in a blender and blend until smooth.
Serve immediately.

Nutritional Information:

Calories: 464
Protein: 26g
Fat: 21g
Carbs: 47g

CHOCOLATE AVOCADO SMOOTHIE

Ingredients:

1 avocado
1 cup almond milk
1 scoop chocolate protein powder
1 tsp honey
1 tsp vanilla extract

Instructions:

Combine all ingredients in a blender and blend until smooth.
Serve immediately.

Nutritional Information:

Calories: 477
Protein: 25g
Fat: 29g
Carbs: 35g

MANGO COCONUT SHAKE

Ingredients:

1 mango

1 cup coconut milk
1 scoop vanilla protein powder
1 tbsp honey
1 tsp vanilla extract

Instructions:

Combine all ingredients in a blender and blend until smooth.
Serve immediately.

Nutritional Information:

Calories: 457
Protein: 23g
Fat: 21g
Carbs: 53g

BLUEBERRY ALMOND BUTTER SMOOTHIE

Ingredients:

1 cup frozen blueberries
1 cup almond milk
2 tbsp almond butter
1 scoop vanilla protein powder
1 tsp honey

Instructions:

Combine all ingredients in a blender and blend until smooth.
Serve immediately.

Nutritional Information:

Calories: 441
Protein: 24g
Fat: 22g
Carbs: 42g

OATMEAL RAISIN COOKIE SHAKE

Ingredients:

1 cup oatmeal
1 banana
1 cup milk
1 scoop vanilla protein powder
1 tbsp raisins
1 tsp cinnamon
1 tsp honey

Instructions:

Combine all ingredients in a blender and blend until smooth.
Serve immediately.

Nutritional Information:

Calories: 525
Protein: 28g
Fat: 11g
Carbs: 85g

NUTELLA BANANA SHAKE

Ingredients:

1 banana
2 tbsp Nutella
1 cup milk
1 scoop chocolate protein powder
1 tsp vanilla extract

Instructions:

Combine all ingredients in a blender and blend until smooth.
Serve immediately.

Nutritional Information:

Calories: 551
Protein: 27g
Fat: 21g

Carbs: 67g

Ingredients:

1 banana
1 tbsp peanut butter
1 tbsp cocoa powder
1 cup milk
1 scoop chocolate protein powder
1 tsp honey

Instructions:

Combine all ingredients in a blender and blend until smooth.
Serve immediately.

Nutritional Information:

Calories: 451
Protein: 31g
Fat: 14g
Carbs: 52g

STRAWBERRY COCONUT SHAKE

Ingredients:

1 cup frozen strawberries
1 cup coconut milk
1 scoop vanilla protein powder
1 tbsp honey
1 tsp vanilla extract

Instructions:

Combine all ingredients in a blender and blend until smooth.
Serve immediately.

Nutritional Information:

Calories: 390
Protein: 21g
Fat: 21g
Carbs: 35g

CINNAMON ROLL SHAKE

Ingredients:

1 cup vanilla ice cream
1 cup milk
1 scoop vanilla protein powder
1 tsp cinnamon

1 tsp vanilla extract

Instructions:

Combine all ingredients in a blender and blend until smooth.
Serve immediately.

Nutritional Information:

Calories: 567
Protein: 29g
Fat: 27g
Carbs: 58g

ALMOND JOY SMOOTHIE

Ingredients:

1 banana
1/4 cup almonds
1/4 cup shredded coconut
1 cup milk
1 scoop chocolate protein powder
1 tsp honey

Instructions:

Combine all ingredients in a blender and blend until smooth.
Serve immediately.

Nutritional Information:

Calories: 567
Protein: 29g
Fat: 27g
Carbs: 58g

BANANA NUT SHAKE

Ingredients:

1 banana
1/4 cup walnuts
1 cup milk
1 scoop vanilla protein powder
1 tsp honey

Instructions:

Combine all ingredient
s in a blender and blend until smooth.
Serve immediately.

Nutritional Information:

Calories: 473
Protein: 26g
Fat: 22g
Carbs: 48g

BLUEBERRY OATMEAL SHAKE

Ingredients:

1/2 cup rolled oats
1 cup milk
1 cup frozen blueberries
1 scoop vanilla protein powder
1 tsp honey

Instructions:

Combine rolled oats and milk in a blender and let sit
for 5-10 minutes.
Add frozen blueberries, vanilla protein powder, and
honey to the blender and blend until smooth.
Serve immediately.

Nutritional Information:

Calories: 466
Protein: 26g
Fat: 8g
Carbs: 74g

AVOCADO MANGO SMOOTHIE

Ingredients:

1/2 avocado
1 cup frozen mango chunks
1 cup coconut milk
1 scoop vanilla protein powder
1 tsp honey

Instructions:

Combine all ingredients in a blender and blend until smooth.
Serve immediately.

Nutritional Information:

Calories: 441
Protein: 22g
Fat: 26g
Carbs: 38g

PEANUT BUTTER CUP SMOOTHIE

Ingredients:

1 banana

1 tbsp peanut butter
1 tbsp cocoa powder
1 cup almond milk
1 scoop chocolate protein powder
1 tsp honey

Instructions:

Combine all ingredients in a blender and blend until smooth.
Serve immediately.

Nutritional information:

Calories: 406
Protein: 24g
Fat: 16g
Carbs: 47g

COCONUT PINEAPPLE SMOOTHIE

Ingredients:

1 cup frozen pineapple chunks
1 cup coconut milk
1 scoop vanilla protein powder
1 tbsp honey
1 tsp vanilla extract

Instructions:

Combine all ingredients in a blender and blend until smooth.
Serve immediately.

Nutritional Information:

Calories: 367
Protein: 21g
Fat: 22g
Carbs: 28g

APPLE CINNAMON OAT SHAKE

Ingredients:

1 apple, cored and sliced
1/2 cup rolled oats
1 cup milk
1 scoop vanilla protein powder
1 tsp honey
1 tsp cinnamon

Instructions:

Combine apple slices, rolled oats, and milk in a blender and let sit for 5-10 minutes.

Add vanilla protein powder, honey, and cinnamon to the blender and blend until smooth.
Serve immediately.

Nutritional Information:

Calories: 448
Protein: 26g
Fat: 9g
Carbs: 68g

CHOCOLATE CHERRY SMOOTHIE

Ingredients:

1 cup frozen cherries
1 cup almond milk
1 scoop chocolate protein powder
1 tbsp cocoa powder
1 tsp honey

Instructions:

Combine all ingredients in a blender and blend until smooth.
Serve immediately.

Nutritional Information:

Calories: 307
Protein: 24g
Fat: 8g
Carbs: 38g

GREEN ENERGY SMOOTHIE

Ingredients:

1 banana
1 cup spinach leaves
1 cup almond milk
1 scoop vanilla protein powder
1 tsp honey
1 tsp chia seeds

Instructions:

Combine all ingredients in a blender and blend until smooth.
Serve immediately.

Nutritional Information:

Calories: 321
Protein: 19g
Fat: 9g
Carbs: 45g

BANANA NUT SMOOTHIE

Ingredients:

1 banana
1/4 cup walnuts
1 cup milk
1 scoop vanilla protein powder
1 tsp honey
1/2 tsp cinnamon

Instructions:

Combine banana, walnuts, and milk in a blender
and let sit for 5-10 minutes.
Add vanilla protein powder, honey, and cinnamon
to the blender and blend until smooth.
Serve immediately.

Nutritional Information:

Calories: 502
Protein: 28g
Fat: 26g
Carbs: 46g

CHAPTER 9

While the best way to gain weight is through a balanced diet and regular exercise, there are some supplements that can aid in weight gain for men. Here are some options:

Whey protein powder: Whey protein is a popular supplement among bodybuilders and fitness enthusiasts as it is an excellent source of protein. Adding whey protein powder to your diet can help increase your protein intake and promote muscle growth.

Creatine: Creatine is a naturally occurring compound in the body that can also be found in supplement form. It can increase muscle mass and strength, making it a popular choice for those looking to bulk up.

Weight gainers: Weight gainers are high-calorie supplements that contain a mix of protein, carbohydrates, and fat. They can help increase your overall calorie intake and support weight gain.

Omega-3 fatty acids: Omega-3 fatty acids are essential fatty acids that play a role in several bodily functions, including muscle growth and repair. They can be found in supplement form or in foods like fatty fish, nuts, and seeds.

Multivitamins: Taking a multivitamin can help ensure that your body is getting all the necessary vitamins and minerals it needs to support weight gain.

It's important to note that supplements should be used in conjunction with a healthy diet and exercise regimen, not as a replacement. It's also important to speak with a healthcare professional before starting any new supplement regimen.

SUPPLEMENTS THAT CAN AID IN WEIGHT GAIN FOR MEN

While weight gain supplements can be helpful in supporting muscle growth and recovery, it's important to remember that they should always be used in combination with a healthy diet and regular exercise program. Here are some supplements that may aid in weight gain for men:

Whey protein: This is a high-quality protein that is easily digested by the body and can help support muscle growth and repair.

Creatine: This supplement is known to increase muscle strength and size by helping to increase energy production in the muscles.

Mass gainers: These are supplements that contain a combination of protein, carbohydrates, and fats to help increase calorie intake and support weight gain.

BCAAs (Branched-Chain Amino Acids): These are essential amino acids that can help support muscle growth and recovery.

Beta-Alanine: This supplement can help increase endurance and improve muscle performance during high-intensity workouts.

Omega-3 fatty acids: These healthy fats can help support overall health and may aid in reducing inflammation in the body.

Glutamine: This is an amino acid that plays a crucial role in muscle recovery and growth. It can help to reduce muscle breakdown and increase protein synthesis, which may aid in building muscle mass. Additionally, it may help to support the immune system and digestive health.

D-Aspartic Acid (DAA): This is an amino acid that has been shown to increase testosterone levels in men, which may aid in muscle growth and recovery. Higher testosterone levels can also help increase energy levels, improve mood, and support overall health. However, it's important to note that DAA should only be taken under the supervision of a healthcare professional, as excessive levels of testosterone can have negative health effects.

HMB (Beta-Hydroxy Beta-Methylbutyrate): This is a metabolite of the amino acid leucine that has been shown to help increase muscle mass and strength, particularly in combination with exercise. It may also aid in reducing muscle damage and fatigue, allowing for faster recovery and improved performance. However, it's important to note that the research on HMB is still limited and more studies are needed to fully understand its effects.

Zinc: This essential mineral is important for overall health and may aid in supporting muscle growth and recovery. Zinc plays a role in protein synthesis and testosterone production, both of which are important for building muscle mass. Additionally, zinc may help support immune function and reduce inflammation in the body. However, it's important not to take too much zinc, as excessive amounts can have negative health effects. It's best to speak with a healthcare professional to determine the appropriate dosage for your needs.

PROS AND CONS OF USING SUPPLEMENT IN WEIGHT GAIN

Using supplements for weight gain can have both advantages and disadvantages. Here are some of the pros and cons:

PROS:

Convenience: Supplements are convenient and easy to use, making them a popular choice for people who have a busy lifestyle or have trouble eating enough food.

Increased calorie intake: Supplements are usually high in calories, which can help you consume more calories than you burn, leading to weight gain.

Nutrient-dense: Many supplements contain vitamins, minerals, and other nutrients that are important for overall health, making them a good option for people who may have nutrient deficiencies.

Variety: There are many different types of supplements available, which can help you find one that fits your specific dietary needs and preferences.

CONS:

Cost: Supplements can be expensive, especially if you are using them on a regular basis.

Safety: Some supplements may contain harmful ingredients or contaminants, which can pose a risk to your health.

Dependence: Using supplements as your primary source of calories can create a dependence on them, making it difficult to meet your nutritional needs without them.

Digestive Issues: Some supplements can cause digestive issues, such as bloating, gas, and diarrhea.

In summary, while supplements can be a useful tool for weight gain, it's important to consider the potential drawbacks and make sure you are using them safely and responsibly. It's always a good idea to consult with a healthcare professional before starting any supplement regimen.

Before taking any supplements to gain weight, it's important to speak with a healthcare professional or a registered dietitian to determine if they are appropriate for your individual needs and goals.

Assuming that you have consulted with a healthcare professional and have determined that weight gain supplements are right for you, the following are general recommendations for dosage and precautions:

Creatine: Creatine is a popular supplement for increasing muscle mass and strength. The recommended dosage is typically 5 grams per day, taken with a meal or after exercise. However, it's important to drink plenty of water while taking creatine, as it can cause dehydration if not consumed with enough fluids.

Protein powder: Protein powder is commonly used to supplement a high-protein diet for muscle growth and repair. The recommended dosage varies depending on the individual's weight and activity level, but generally ranges from 20-30 grams per serving. It's important to choose a high-quality protein powder and to avoid consuming excessive amounts of protein, as this can strain the kidneys.

Weight gainers: Weight gainers are supplements designed to provide a high calorie intake in order to promote weight gain. The recommended dosage varies depending on the product, but typically ranges from 500-1000 calories per serving. It's important to read the label carefully and choose a weight gainer that provides high-quality ingredients and does not contain excessive amounts of sugar or unhealthy fats.

Precautions: It's important to remember that supplements are not a substitute for a healthy diet and exercise routine. Taking excessive amounts of supplements can have negative effects on your health, and some supplements may interact with medications or have negative side effects. Always speak with a healthcare professional before beginning any supplement regimen, and carefully read the label to ensure you are taking the proper dosage and following all precautions.

Safety: It's important to purchase supplements from reputable brands that are certified by third-party organizations such as the United States Pharmacopeia (USP), NSF International, or ConsumerLab. This can help ensure that the supplements are free from contaminants and accurately labeled. Additionally, always follow the instructions and recommended dosages on the label and store supplements in a cool, dry place away from children and pets. If you experience any negative side effects while taking a supplement, discontinue use and speak with a healthcare professional.

In addition to following recommended dosages, it is important to take supplements with food and to drink plenty of water to prevent dehydration. It is also important to be aware of any potential interactions with medications or other supplements that you may be taking. Finally, it is important to remember that supplements should not replace a healthy diet and exercise regimen for weight gain.

CHAPTER 10

To gain weight, it's important to focus on strength training exercises that help build muscle mass. Here are some exercises that can help men gain weight:

Squats: Squats are a compound exercise that work the muscles in the legs, hips, and glutes. They are one of the most effective exercises for building muscle mass.

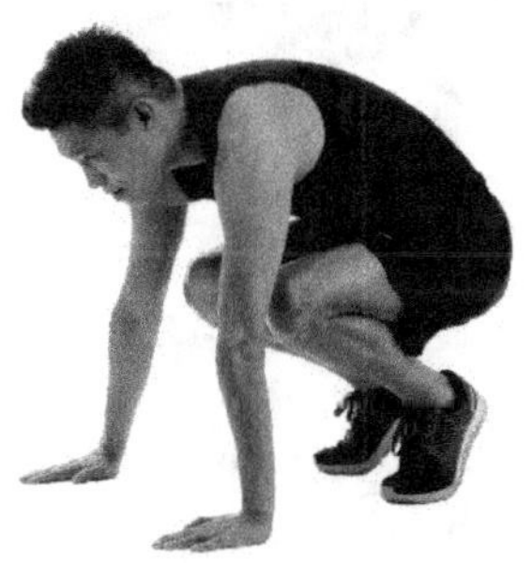

Deadlifts: Deadlifts work multiple muscle groups, including the back, legs, and core. They are great for building overall strength and muscle mass.

Bench Press: The bench press is an effective exercise for building chest, shoulder, and tricep muscles.

Barbell Rows: Barbell rows work the muscles in the back and can help build overall upper body strength.

Pull-Ups: Pull-ups are a bodyweight exercise that work the muscles in the back, shoulders, and arms. They can help build upper body strength and muscle mass.

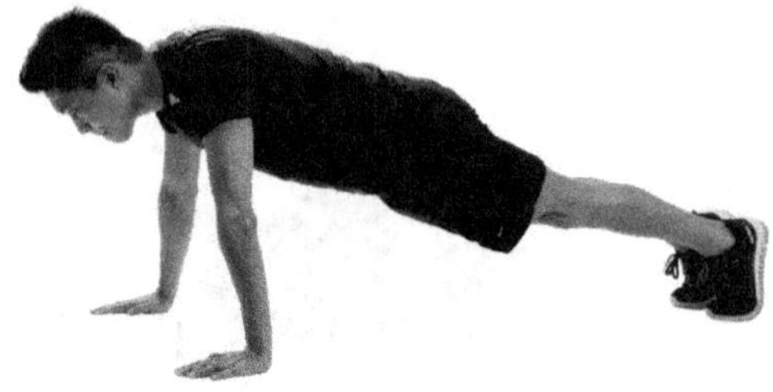

Overhead Press: The overhead press works the muscles in the shoulders and can help build upper body strength.

Bicep Curls: Bicep curls target the muscles in the arms and can help build arm strength and muscle mass.

Lunges: Lunges are a compound exercise that work the muscles in the legs, hips, and glutes. They can help build lower body strength and muscle mass.

Dumbbell Flys: Dumbbell flys are a great exercise for building chest muscles. They target the pectoral muscles and help to create a wider and fuller chest.

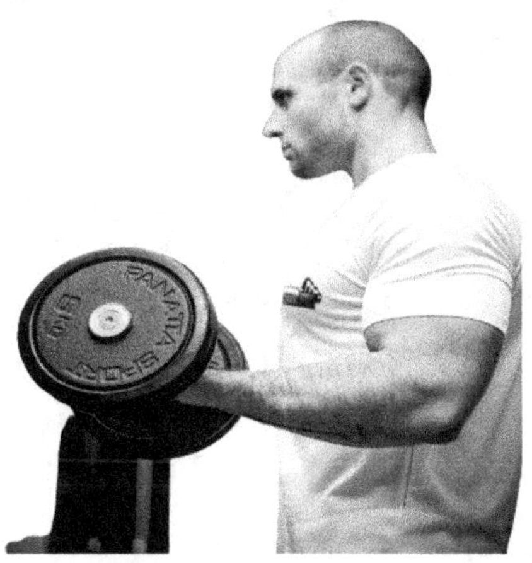

Tricep Extensions: Tricep extensions work the muscles in the back of the arms and can help build arm strength and muscle mass.

Calf Raises: Calf raises are a great exercise for building the muscles in the lower legs. They can help to create a more defined and sculpted appearance in the calves.

Incline Dumbbell Press: Incline dumbbell press is a variation of the bench press that targets the upper chest muscles. This exercise can help to create a more defined and sculpted chest.

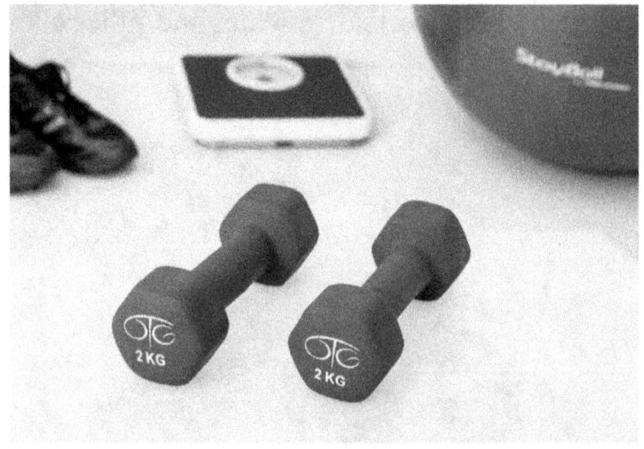

Remember to always use proper form when performing these exercises to avoid injury and consult with a trainer or healthcare professional if you are new to weightlifting.

It's important to note that while exercise is important for building muscle mass, it's also essential to consume enough calories and protein to support muscle growth, that is where the recipes in this book comes in handy.

Additionally, make sure to rest and allow your muscles to recover between workouts to avoid injury and promote optimal muscle growth.

TIPS AND TRICKS FOR LONG-TERM SUCCESS FOR WEIGHT GAIN AND LIFESTYLE CHANGES TO SUPPORT WEIGHT GAIN FOR MEN

Weight gain can be just as challenging as weight loss, especially for men who want to bulk up and build muscle mass. Here are some tips and tricks that can help you successfully gain weight:

Increase your calorie intake: To gain weight, you need to consume more calories than you burn. Calculate your daily calorie needs using an online calculator, and aim to consume 500 to 1,000 calories more than that.

Focus on nutrient-dense foods: Choose foods that are high in protein, healthy fats, and complex carbohydrates, such as whole grains, nuts, seeds, lean meats, fish, and dairy products.

Eat frequently: Instead of three large meals a day, aim to eat five to six smaller meals throughout the day to keep your metabolism active and provide your body with a steady supply of nutrients.

Strength train: Incorporate strength training exercises into your workout routine to build muscle mass. Focus on compound exercises, such as squats, deadlifts, and bench presses, which work multiple muscle groups at once.

Lift weights: Resistance training is an effective way to build muscle mass. Incorporate weightlifting exercises into your workout routine to stimulate muscle growth.

Get enough rest: Adequate rest and recovery time is crucial for muscle growth. Aim for 7 to 9 hours of sleep each night and avoid overtraining.

Track your progress: Keep a record of your weight, body measurements, and workout progress to track your progress and make adjustments to your diet and exercise routine as needed. To make tracking your progress easier, you can also get my weight gain tracker book.

Consider supplements: Supplements such as protein powder, creatine, and weight gainers can be helpful in providing your body with the extra nutrients it needs to build muscle mass. However, always consult with a healthcare professional before taking any supplements.

Stay hydrated: Drinking enough water is important for overall health and can help support muscle growth. Aim to drink at least 8 to 10 glasses of water per day, and more if you're engaging in strenuous exercise or sweating excessively. Dehydration can negatively impact muscle growth and recovery.

Avoid smoking and excessive alcohol consumption: These habits can negatively impact your weight gain goals.

Remember, weight gain is a gradual process, and it may take several months to see significant results. Consistency, patience, and dedication are key to achieving your weight gain goals.

DEALING WITH CHALLENGES AND SETBACKS IN WEIGHT GAIN FOR MEN

Gaining weight can be a challenging process for some men, and setbacks can often occur along the way. Here are some tips for dealing with challenges and setbacks in weight gain:

Set realistic goals: It's important to set realistic goals when it comes to weight gain. Aim to gain no more than 1-2 pounds per week, as gaining weight too quickly can lead to health problems.

Track your progress: Keep track of your weight gain progress by regularly weighing yourself and taking measurements. This can help you identify any plateaus or setbacks and adjust your approach accordingly.

Eat a balanced diet: Focus on consuming a balanced diet that includes plenty of protein, complex carbohydrates, and healthy fats. This will help provide your body with the nutrients it needs to build muscle and gain weight.

Incorporate strength training: Strength training is crucial for gaining muscle mass and weight. Make sure to incorporate exercises that target all major muscle groups, and gradually increase the weight and intensity of your workouts over time.

Get enough rest: Adequate rest is essential for muscle recovery and growth. Aim to get 7-8 hours of sleep each night, and take rest days between workouts to allow your muscles time to repair and rebuild.

Stay motivated: It's important to stay motivated and focused on your goals, even when setbacks occur. Find a workout partner, keep a progress journal, or reward yourself for reaching milestones to help stay motivated.

Be patient: Gaining weight takes time and effort, and setbacks are a natural part of the process. Don't get discouraged if progress seems slow or if you experience setbacks along the way. Stay committed to your goals and keep working towards them, and you'll eventually see the results you're looking for.

Identify the cause of setbacks: If you experience setbacks in your weight gain journey, take some time to identify the cause. Maybe you've been consuming too many processed foods or skipping workouts. Once you identify the cause, you can make necessary adjustments to your diet or exercise routine to get back on track.

Stay consistent: Consistency is key when it comes to gaining weight. Make sure to stick to your diet and exercise plan, even when you're not seeing immediate results. Consistency over time will help you reach your goals and avoid setbacks.

Don't compare yourself to others: It's important to remember that everyone's weight gain journey is unique. Avoid comparing yourself to others, as this can lead to feelings of discouragement or frustration. Focus on your own progress and celebrate your own achievements.

Stay hydrated: Drinking plenty of water is important for overall health and can also help with weight gain. Aim to drink at least 8-10 glasses of water per day, and consider adding in other hydrating beverages like coconut water or sports drinks to help replenish electrolytes lost during workouts.

Seek professional help: If you're struggling to gain weight or experiencing setbacks, consider seeking the help of a nutritionist or personal trainer. They can provide guidance and support to help you reach your goals.

HOW TO MEASURE PROGRESS AND ADJUST YOUR DIET

To measure progress and adjust your diet for weight gain, men should consider the following steps:

Calculate your daily caloric needs: To gain weight, you need to consume more calories than you burn each day. You can use online calculators or consult a nutritionist to determine your daily caloric needs based on your age, height, weight, and activity level.

Track your calorie intake: Use a food diary or an app to track what you eat and drink each day. This will help you determine if you are consuming enough calories to gain weight.

Monitor your weight: Weigh yourself regularly to track your progress. Aim to gain 0.5 to 1 pound per week.

Adjust your diet: If you are not gaining weight, you may need to increase your calorie intake. Add more healthy, high-calorie foods to your diet such as nuts, seeds, avocados, whole-grain bread, and pasta. Try to eat more frequently throughout the day and increase your portion sizes.

Keep protein intake high: To build muscle mass, men need to consume adequate protein. Aim to consume at least 1 gram of protein per pound of body weight each day.

Incorporate strength training: Along with a high-calorie diet, strength training is crucial for gaining muscle mass. Focus on compound exercises such as squats, deadlifts, and bench press.

Be patient: Gaining weight and building muscle takes time, so be patient and consistent with your diet and exercise routine.

Keep track of your progress: Continuously monitor your progress by tracking your weight, body measurements, and strength gains. This will help you make adjustments to your diet and exercise routine as needed.

I have made tracking your weight gain a lot easier you can get my book on weight tracking to begin the track record of your days to a healthy weight gain.

Stay consistent: Consistency is key when it comes to weight gain. Stick to your meal plan and exercise routine, even on days when you don't feel motivated. Over time, your hard work will pay off with visible results.

CHAPTER 11

CONCLUSION AND NEXT STEPS

Conclusion:

In conclusion, gaining weight requires a strategic approach to nutrition and exercise. This weight gain diet cookbook for men is a useful resource for men who want to gain weight in a healthy and sustainable way. This cookbook provides a variety of recipes that are high in calories, protein, and healthy fats, which are essential for building muscle and gaining weight.

By following the recipes in this cookbook and incorporating them into a well-rounded diet and exercise plan, men can achieve their weight gain goals.

Next Steps:

To maximize the benefits of this weight gain diet cookbook, men should consider the following next steps:

Consult with a healthcare professional or a registered dietitian to determine their individualized caloric and nutritional needs.

Use the recipes in the cookbook as a starting point and modify them based on personal preferences and dietary restrictions.

Incorporate other healthy foods and snacks into their diet to ensure they are meeting all of their nutritional needs.

Combine a healthy diet with a regular exercise routine that includes both strength training and cardio to build muscle and improve overall health.

Monitor progress regularly and make adjustments to the diet and exercise plan as needed to achieve weight gain goals.

APPENDIX

Weight gain for men can be influenced by a variety of factors, including genetics, diet, exercise habits, and overall lifestyle. Here are some additional pieces of information on weight gain for men:

Calorie intake: Men generally have higher calorie requirements than women due to their higher muscle mass and generally larger body size. Consuming more calories than your body needs can lead to weight gain.

Muscle mass: Men have more muscle mass than women on average, which can impact weight gain. Building muscle through strength training can increase overall body weight, but can also lead to a more toned and muscular physique.

Age: Men tend to experience a decline in metabolism and muscle mass as they age, which can lead to weight gain if dietary and exercise habits do not adjust accordingly.

Hormones: Testosterone plays a role in muscle growth and weight gain in men. Low testosterone levels may contribute to weight gain and difficulty losing weight.

Sleep: Poor sleep habits can contribute to weight gain in men. Lack of sleep can disrupt hormone levels, including those that regulate appetite and metabolism.

Stress: Chronic stress can lead to weight gain due to increased cortisol levels. Cortisol is a hormone that is released in response to stress and can contribute to increased appetite and fat storage.

Genetics: Genetics can influence body weight and fat distribution. Some men may have a genetic predisposition to weight gain or difficulty losing weight.

Alcohol consumption: Drinking alcohol can contribute to weight gain in men. Alcoholic beverages are high in calories and can lead to increased appetite and decreased inhibitions, leading to overeating or making poor food choices. Additionally, excessive alcohol consumption can damage the liver, which plays a role in metabolism and fat storage. Cutting back on alcohol or avoiding it altogether can help with weight management.

Sedentary lifestyle: Lack of physical activity can contribute to weight gain in men. Regular exercise helps to burn calories and build muscle mass, which can increase metabolism and aid in weight management. Men who have jobs that require sitting for long periods of time should make an effort to incorporate physical activity into their daily routine, such as taking regular breaks to stand up and stretch or going for a walk during lunch breaks.

Medical conditions: Certain medical conditions can contribute to weight gain in men. For example, hypothyroidism, a condition in which the thyroid gland doesn't produce enough thyroid hormone, can cause weight gain and difficulty losing weight. Other conditions such as Cushing's syndrome, polycystic ovary syndrome (PCOS), and sleep apnea can also contribute to weight gain. If you're experiencing unexplained weight gain, it's important to talk to a healthcare professional to rule out any underlying medical conditions.

It's important to note that healthy weight gain should involve a combination of increasing muscle mass and consuming a healthy, balanced diet that provides enough calories to support growth and development. It's always a good idea to consult with a healthcare professional or registered dietitian to determine the best approach for your individual needs.

GLOSSARY OF TERMS

Weight gain: The increase in body weight over time.

Body mass index (BMI): A measure of body fat based on height and weight. A BMI of 25 or higher is considered overweight, while a BMI of 30 or higher is considered obese.

Lean body mass: The weight of the body without its fat content.

Fat mass: The amount of fat in the body.

Calorie: A unit of energy, usually used to measure the energy content of food.

Caloric surplus: A situation where an individual consumes more calories than they burn, resulting in weight gain.

Basal metabolic rate (BMR): The amount of energy the body uses at rest to maintain basic bodily functions such as breathing and circulation.

Muscle hypertrophy: The growth and increase in size of muscle fibers.

Resistance training: A type of exercise that involves working against a resistance to build strength and muscle.

Bulking: A period of time where an individual intentionally increases their caloric intake and engages in resistance training to gain muscle mass.

Overfeeding: A dietary practice where an individual consumes more calories than their body needs, resulting in weight gain.

Resting metabolic rate (RMR): The amount of energy the body uses at rest to maintain basic bodily functions such as breathing and circulation.

Anabolic: A state where the body is building or repairing tissue, such as muscle.

Catabolic: A state where the body is breaking down tissue, such as muscle.

Macronutrients: Nutrients required in large amounts in the diet, including carbohydrates, proteins, and fats.

Micronutrients: Nutrients required in small amounts in the diet, including vitamins and minerals.

Testosterone: A hormone produced by the testicles that plays a crucial role in the development of male reproductive tissues and secondary sexual characteristics. Testosterone also helps to build muscle and bone mass.

Growth hormone: A hormone produced by the pituitary gland that stimulates growth, cell reproduction, and regeneration in humans and other animals. Growth hormone also plays a role in building muscle mass.

Insulin: A hormone produced by the pancreas that regulates blood sugar levels by facilitating the absorption of glucose into cells. Insulin also promotes the storage of excess calories as fat.

Metabolism: The chemical processes that occur in the body to maintain life. Metabolism includes the conversion of food into energy and the elimination of waste products.

Thermogenesis: The process of heat production in the body. Thermogenesis can increase energy expenditure and help to burn calories.

Adipose tissue: A type of connective tissue that stores fat in the body. Adipose tissue also produces hormones that regulate metabolism.

Cortisol: A hormone produced by the adrenal gland in response to stress. Cortisol can increase appetite and promote the storage of fat in the body.

Leptin: A hormone produced by fat cells that regulates appetite and energy expenditure. Leptin signals the brain when the body has had enough to eat and can help to prevent overeating.

Ghrelin: A hormone produced in the stomach that stimulates appetite. Ghrelin levels increase before meals and decrease after meals.

Satiety: The feeling of fullness and satisfaction after a meal that suppresses hunger and reduces the desire to eat.

Nutrient timing: The practice of consuming specific nutrients at specific times to optimize muscle growth and recovery.

Protein synthesis: The process by which cells build proteins. Protein synthesis is important for muscle growth and repair.

Rest and recovery: The period of time after exercise when the body repairs and rebuilds muscle tissue.

Rest and recovery are essential for muscle growth and preventing injury.

Progressive overload: The gradual increase in the intensity, volume, or frequency of exercise to stimulate muscle growth and prevent a plateau in results.

Macronutrient ratio: The proportion of carbohydrates, proteins, and fats in the diet. The optimal macronutrient ratio for weight gain may vary depending on individual factors such as age, sex, and activity level.

Fiber: A type of carbohydrate that the body cannot digest. Fiber helps to regulate digestion and can promote feelings of fullness.

Trans fats: A type of fat that is often found in processed foods. Trans fats can raise cholesterol levels and increase the risk of heart disease.

Omega-3 fatty acids: A type of polyunsaturated fat that is found in fish, nuts, and seeds. Omega-3 fatty acids have anti-inflammatory properties and can help to reduce the risk of heart disease.

Omega-6 fatty acids: A type of polyunsaturated fat that is found in vegetable oils and processed foods.

Omega-6 fatty acids are important for overall health but can be harmful in excess.

Water weight: The temporary increase in body weight due to water retention. Water weight can be caused by factors such as a high-sodium diet, hormonal changes, or dehydration.

Body recomposition: The process of changing body composition by simultaneously reducing body fat and building muscle mass.

Resting heart rate (RHR): The number of times the heart beats per minute while at rest. RHR can be used as an indicator of overall cardiovascular health and fitness.

High-intensity interval training (HIIT): A type of exercise that involves short bursts of intense activity followed by periods of rest or lower-intensity exercise. HIIT can help to increase metabolism and promote fat loss.

Cardiovascular exercise: Exercise that involves sustained physical activity that raises the heart rate and improves cardiovascular health. Examples include running, cycling, and swimming.

Anabolic window: The period of time after exercise when the body is most receptive to protein and carbohydrate consumption to optimize muscle growth and recovery.

Bodybuilding: A sport that involves the use of resistance training and diet to increase muscle size and improve overall physique.

Powerlifting: A strength sport that involves three main lifts: squat, bench press, and deadlift.

Crossfit: A fitness program that combines various types of exercise, including weightlifting, cardiovascular exercise, and gymnastics.

Fitness plateau: A point at which progress in physical fitness or weight gain stalls despite continued effort. A plateau can be overcome by changing up the exercise routine or adjusting the diet.

Bulking: A phase of weight training during which a person increases their caloric intake to gain muscle mass and strength.

Cutting: A phase of weight training during which a person reduces their caloric intake to lose body fat while maintaining muscle mass.

Body mass index (BMI): A measure of body fat based on height and weight. BMI can be used as an indicator of overall health and fitness, but it has limitations and may not be accurate for individuals with a high level of muscle mass.

Body fat percentage: The percentage of body weight that is made up of fat. Body fat percentage can be measured using various methods, such as skinfold calipers or bioelectrical impedance analysis.

Calorie surplus: A state in which a person consumes more calories than they burn, leading to weight gain.

Calorie deficit: A state in which a person burns more calories than they consume, leading to weight loss.

Clean eating: A dietary approach that emphasizes whole, minimally processed foods and avoids added sugars, trans fats, and other unhealthy ingredients.

Cheat meal: A meal or snack that is consumed outside of a person's usual dietary regimen. Cheat meals are often used as a reward for sticking to a healthy diet.

Macronutrient tracking: The practice of monitoring and adjusting the intake of carbohydrates, proteins, and fats to achieve specific dietary goals.

Supplement: A product that is taken in addition to a person's normal diet to provide specific nutrients or enhance athletic performance. Supplements may include vitamins, minerals, protein powders, or pre-workout formulas.

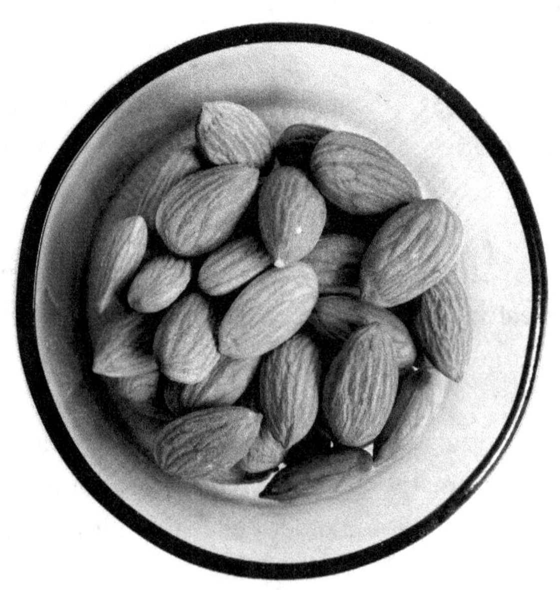

RECOMMENDED WEBSITES

Bodybuilding.com - This website offers a wide range of articles, tips, and workout plans for men who want to gain weight and build muscle.

Men's Health - Men's Health provides articles, recipes, and workout plans specifically tailored for men looking to gain weight and build muscle.

Muscle and Fitness - This website provides workout plans, nutrition tips, and supplement recommendations for men who want to gain muscle mass and increase their weight.

GainingWeight.info - This website offers information and advice on how to gain weight through diet and exercise.

WeightGainPro.com - WeightGainPro.com provides articles, tips, and workout plans for men looking to gain weight, build muscle, and improve their overall health and fitness.

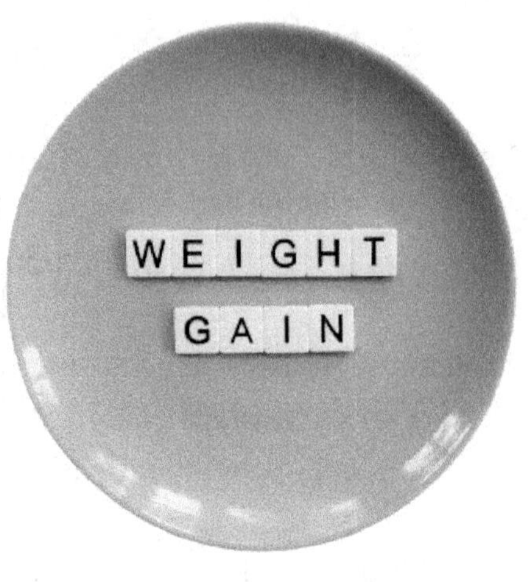

WEIGHT
GAIN